"Coco's 'Confessions of a Diet Junkie' alone is worth the price of the book."

—Elizabeth Lay,
San Francisco Chronicle

"I must say his book is the most sensible one in the genre."

—Liz Smith,
Syndicated Columnist

Finally, I was in control of my own destiny . . .

Once I mastered the diet program, I began to adapt it to what worked best for me. I began to experiment and to invent my own recipes—and the more I experimented the better I got. Everybody loves my veal loaf. I serve it with peppers and roasted potatoes garnished with parsley. By candlelight. It is a structured meal. *People* magazine featured it in one issue. I have learned a lot about myself, my phobias and anxieties, my hang-ups and my own historical reasons for overeating. A lot of things I was afraid to ask myself I asked myself. There is no magic pill. But there are answers. The stresses may never disappear—but I have the tools, the techniques, and the knowledge and determination to overcome them. I will probably always have to struggle, but I will win. And if I can, you can!

—JAMES COCO

The James Coco Diet

James Coco

with Marion Paone

BANTAM BOOKS
TORONTO · NEW YORK · LONDON · SYDNEY · AUCKLAND

Caution: *Before starting any diet you should consult your doctor to discuss the reducing plan you intend to follow.*

THE JAMES COCO DIET

Bantam Hardcover edition / February 1984
9 printings through April 1984
Bantam rack-size edition / February 1985

Grateful acknowledgment is made to Rex Reed for his permission to quote from Valentines & Vitriol *copyright © 1977 by Rex Reed. All rights reserved.*

Library of Congress Cataloging in Publication Data

Coco, James.
    The James Coco diet.

    Includes index.
    1. Low-calorie diet. 2. Low-calorie diet—Recipes.
3. Food—Calorie content—Tables. I. Paone, Marion.
II. Title.
RM222.2.C54   1984   613.2'5   83-22344
ISBN 0-553-24514-7

Published simultaneously in the United States and Canada

PRINTED IN THE UNITED STATES OF AMERICA

O   0 9 8 7 6 5 4 3 2 1

This book is dedicated to
Lucia Coco Negri and
Nellie Paone, for all the obvious reasons

Contents

Acknowledgments

In her acceptance speech at the 1981 Academy Award ceremonies, Maureen Stapleton, honored for her performance in the movie, *Reds,* concluded by saying, "and I would like to thank everybody I have ever met in my entire life." I now know how she felt. Finishing a book is also a time for thank yous. So many people have helped in so many different ways: some, by just being there like family and friends; others, in more tangible ways. To name a few; Structure House, for allowing us to use some of their recipes and for their invaluable assistance with the chapter on behavior modification. Pat Andrews, Structure House nutritionist who trekked from North Carolina to New York at a moment's notice (and none too soon) to help with the chapter, "Nutrition: A Drama in One Act"; Dr. Siegfried H. Heyden, professor of community health sciences at the Duke University Medical Center and pioneer in the science of weight control who enthusiastically shared with us his vast knowledge of the subject; Dr. Alfred J. Siegman, who kept on trying when the going got very rough; Marian Rayne, who was always there with the right word; Professor Fred Collins at Memphis State, Tennessee, confidante, mentor, and friend; Jay Garon, our literary agent and friend who opened the door for us; and finally, Brad Miner, our editor, whose guidance and expertise were only surpassed by his enthusiasm and support during the entire writing of this book.

Author's Preface

If you are reading this book to find out what Johnny Carson is really like, or if Joan Rivers is as funny off camera as she is on, keep reading—you just might.

You will also find out what it took me seven years to learn—how to diet the right way. I probably hold the world record for dieting. I have tried them all: The Pregnant Women's Urine Diet, The Water Diet, The Banana and Cream Diet, The No Fat Diet, The All Fat Diet, The Liquid Diet, The Eggs Diet and even the No Eating or Drinking *Anything* Diet, and one that I think is called the Total Starvation Diet.

You have probably tried some or all of the above yourself. Maybe even a few I haven't tried. But one thing I'm sure of—like me, you failed! Believe me, I know how frustrating it is to be on that roller coaster. I also know how dangerous it is to your health. This book is a way *off* the roller coaster for good.

Everybody loves a winner. I want my book to make you a winner by making you a "loser."

I have always loved to eat, and I still love to eat, but *now* I know how to eat, when to eat, and what to eat. The facts are all here—everything you need and *must* know about nutrition and behavior modification; about how emotional stress affects your diet and what to do about it; about the importance of knowing how to read labels; and about how the Structure House program in Durham, North Carolina, works and how to apply it in your own home. How to deal with restaurant dining, dinner parties, and many other important and vital facts are also included.

There is a 21-day diet plan that is easy to follow and gets terrific results, and there are mouth-watering recipes that your friends will swear are fattening.

Most diets are for the birds. My diet is for human beings who love to eat.

You might even find out what Sophia Loren and Raquel Welch are really like, but most importantly, you will find out how to succeed in losing weight, the right way.

Remember—if I can, you can.

JAMES COCO
NEW YORK, NEW YORK
JANUARY 1984

Introduction

by Gerard J. Musante, Ph.D., Director of Structure House

America is overweight. Two out of every five American adults are overweight. In a survey conducted by the National Center for Health Statistics from 1971 to 1974, it was found that the average weight for men and women under age 45 had increased from the previous decade. (The survey also revealed that weight gain occurs most rapidly for women until they are between the ages of 35 and 44; men gain most rapidly until they are between 25 and 34. Both sexes continue to increase weight throughout the later years.)

Attempts to lose weight usually fail. It has been suggested that the cure rate for cancer is greater. It is generally estimated that *only 5 percent of those who lose significant amounts of weight keep it off.*

In spite of these discouraging data, the number of methods for dealing with this problem is truly astounding. Researchers at Johns Hopkins School of Medicine tabulated more than 29,000 theories, treatments, and outright schemes for losing weight over a ten-year period. One million people in the United States participate in various self-help group weight loss programs each week while 9.5 million people go on diets each year. Another 16.5 million are watching their weight so as not to gain, while 26.1 million people have indicated concern for their waistline. The diet food industry booms while appetite suppressants sell at the rate of 80 million dollars a year.

If being overweight is so common, why do we view it in such a negative way and make so many efforts to control it?

Obesity is associated with over 25 known medical conditions. A U.S. Senate Committee estimated that these diseases could account for 15 to 20 percent of all deaths. The "silent killers"—chronic diseases that afflict or will afflict the great majority of us—are strongly linked to obesity. Heart disease, hypertension, diabetes, arthritis, and certain forms of cancer are exacerbated by—if not directly linked to—obesity. Obesity creates a dangerous situation for patients during and after surgery, and many surgeons will not put the obese patient through the risk of surgery unless an emergency arises.

The depression and withdrawal which accompany obesity compound the problem. The frustration of feeling out of control, the anxiety produced by chronic dieting (and regaining) are stresses which further affect the overweight person's medical and mental health. The social stigma attached to obesity affects the overweight person's ability to gain entrance to college and employment.

The economic impact of overweight is staggering. The medical expense of treating obesity-related conditions runs into the billions of dollars.

Furthermore, though Americans spend several billion dollars annually in efforts to lose weight, most dieting schemes and products are fraudulent; many are known to be extremely hazardous. The desperation which leads people to invest their time and money in futile attempts to lose weight seems to deepen as each successive try fails.

How can the problem be solved? The answer is already known. People with obesity of varying degrees of severity and duration have achieved weight control by selecting an approach that is systematic and is based upon *personal* experience rather than upon narrowly defined rules of behavior. All too often professionals, researchers, and practitioners alike begin with a pet theory containing many "do's" and "don't's" that they attempt to impose upon the overweight individual. They seldom observe the individual to see how he responds to various interventions.

I have had the opportunity to work with thousands of overweight people, from 18 to 80 years of age, usually after they have experienced decades of struggle and countless efforts to control weight. I have watched people learn to control their weight by learning to listen to themselves and to understand their own behavior and feelings. This book shows how a person can move in that direction.

Obesity is a very personal problem, different for every single individual. Effective treatment generally is intensive and complex, mirroring the intensity and complexity of the problem itself.

This book will show you that there is no single way to accomplish weight control. There are basic principles, to be sure, but the basic framework is useful only when applied to an individual's personal history and life situation. There is no magic cure. There are clear and definable reasons behind obesity; it is not a mystical curse. By reading this book, everyone can learn how to track and recognize that *they are overeating*. By applying the concepts of *structured eating* and *unstructured eating* they can find out *when* they are overeating. By using the framework of *antecedents,* they can discover *why* they are overeating. In doing so, they can stop searching for the secret reasons and secret cures, and realize that weight control is an ongoing, lifelong process that they, themselves, make happen.

The Structure House program works because it addresses the problems which lead to overeating. It not only helps the person lose weight, but it teaches the person how to keep it off when he or she returns home.

This comprehensive treatment involves a number of factors which are keys to its success. People leave their home environments to come to Structure House. In effect, they are removing themselves from the environment, situations, and people which have a direct influence on their overeating. By staying in the Durham (North Carolina) center, they place themselves in a positive, supportive atmosphere where they see that it is possible to achieve a healthier lifestyle. They actually *live* a healthier lifestyle, learning that they are not compelled by nature to abuse their bodies. The home-like surroundings at Structure House create a comfortable, relaxed feeling which is very important, yet the food and calories are controlled so that weight loss is accomplished easily and consistently. People experience this place as a trusting, open environment where they can recognize the extent of their eating problem and most importantly, readily *admit* to it. In this environment, they begin to realize that weight is primarily a psychological rather than a physiological problem. During the course of treatment, they are taught to identify problems in the three major areas which determine weight: nutrition, exercise, and lifestyle. People can see exactly *when* they turn to food and thus begin to understand *why* they turn to food. Once the problems are identified, they learn specific problem-solving techniques which can be applied immediately. They also begin to map out specific plans for dealing with these problems for application when they return home. By applying the concrete steps which we teach, they recognize that they must face issues and decide what to do about them. They learn that they do have control over these psychological problems. Furthermore, people learn how *to maintain* their weight loss from day one at Structure House. In time, they understand the reasons behind their excess weight, and they come to make a decision whether or not they really *want* to control the problem. Obviously, this book cannot duplicate a visit to Structure House, but this is not a weakness. All of our principles are here. It is simply required of the reader that he or she bring self-discipline to the book.

The Structure House program differs from other diet programs in many ways. It is the only residential obesity treatment program in the country which has a psychological base. Nutrition education, exercise training, and lifestyle counseling are very important parts of the program, but it is the psychological therapy, accomplished within the supportive atmosphere of Structure House itself which helps the individual motivate himself to make use of the tools which the program provides. It is therefore seen as the primary moving force of the program which helps the individual create change in his life.

Other programs fail for a number of reasons. Most are lacking an essential element of thorough treatment. A program may be centered on a faddish, unbalanced diet which is itself unhealthy and unrealistic for use over long periods of time. The program may emphasize exercise in an unhealthy and unrealistic way. Another program might use a sound nutrition and/or exercise plan, but may not address the underlying causes of overeating; the desire to overeat returns unexpectedly after the weight is lost. Others may realize that all these components are important, yet they may not integrate them with the counseling and education necessary to make major lifestyle changes.

Structure House provides all the essential elements and integrates them in a cohesive, understandable program which people can apply individually, both at Structure House and at home.

Because of this approach, Structure House's published results (based on long-term follow-up) are unsurpassed in the field of obesity treatment.

Structure House had its origin in 1977 and was a continuation of my work begun at Duke University five years earlier. From the beginning in 1972, my intention was to combine relevant research with my observation of *individual* patients. From what I had seen, it was difficult to believe that the cause of obesity was as physiological as so many of my physician colleagues had indicated. The realization came about after seeing that once I had developed an individual's trust, he or she was quick to tell me about the large amounts of food consumed. *It was the overeating which led to being overweight.* We were not dealing with a medical cause related to errors of metabolism, but with a behavioral cause related to the desire to overeat in specific situations.

I often saw panic behavior. Large quantities of food would be consumed in extremely short periods of time. Much of the eating/dieting behavior appeared to be extreme. If I were to develop a successful approach to weight loss, I needed a means by which I could determine if there were clear and identifiable external *reasons* why people ate. If I could observe these reasons, it would be much more likely that we were indeed dealing with a psychological rather than a physiological cause to the overeating.

As I began to develop a program in 1972, I realized that many overweight people see themselves in a very negative light; they are guilt-ridden and accustomed to criticism because of their problem. I saw that they needed to develop positive, guilt-free feelings about themselves before they could experience an increased desire to solve their problem.

People had to learn that weight control was not related to

"dieting," but to an ongoing process which involved understanding why food is so important to them. They needed to
change their *attitudes* about losing weight.

People need a sense of control over their eating. After
working with countless individuals, I recognized that eating
is always done for *specific* reasons. At first my patients could
not accept that overeating was willful and done with reason.
Overeating is one of the most complex behavioral and psychological problems to treat. It is typically seen as being
beyond control, compulsive. My observations began to sug-
gest a model for overeating which is circular in nature. I call
this the "vicious cycle"; people often experience eating as
uncontrollable because of its circular nature.

This cycle is developed in the following manner:

- Overeating leads to overweight.
- Simultaneously, as weight increases, individuals cannot
  and do not engage in various activities (as a result of
  increasing physical limitations and the desire to withdraw
  socially).
- A host of negative and self-deprecating internal emotions
  and attitudes are developed over this increasingly un-
  pleasant state.
- In an effort to deal with this emotional, physical, and
  cognitive pain, food is sought as a refuge because 1) it is
  customary (habit-forming); 2) it fills a void; 3) it reduces
  anxiety.

The cycle is thus completed and begins again.

Recognizing this, I needed a way to identify the reasons
for eating and to help people see this for themselves. Of
course, one reason to eat is basic nourishment, that is, in
order for the body to survive—but there are other reasons.
I determined that people needed to *structure* food intake in a
way that enabled them to make the distinction. Structured
eating was to be thought of as that eating necessary for
survival and eventually to maintain one's weight at a desired
level. All other eating that was done had to be considered
unstructured eating, which was done for reasons other than
nourishment.

I devised a special diary for my patients that allowed food

intake to be divided into structured eating on one side and unstructured eating on the other. It was important to develop positive relationships with my patients so that they could feel comfortable in admitting to unstructured eating when it took place. In so doing, I had the opportunity to review diaries which showed episodes of unstructured eating over periods of many months. Gradually, I began to collect the necessary data to determine the reasons underlying unstructured eating. Each episode was painstakingly analyzed with each patient, sorting out the circumstances surrounding this eating, making an effort to identify *antecedents*— that is *cues* that led to the behavior of unstructured eating. Gradually, patterns emerged, ones that proved to be consistent and identifiable. Clear, external situations (antecedents) occurred each and every time, which precipitated the unstructured eating. The conclusion was inevitable. Excess weight was not a medical or physiological problem but a psychological one. I had found a way to have people know *when* they turned to food for nonnutritional, psychological reasons.

The next step was to determine *why* these episodes occurred. As each of these situations was analyzed, specific categories of antecedents emerged. I had reached a startling conclusion. Out of the maze of wondering what overeating was all about, three specific antecedents emerged consistently as precipitating unstructured eating:

Habit: an almost unconscious automatic chain of behaviors learned from earlier childhood by repetition and usually modeled after the behavior of parents and others.

Boredom: using food as entertainment, joy, fun, to fill an otherwise unbearable time void; a pattern that naturally thin people can experience on occasion.

Stress: using food as a tranquilizer when upset, a use of food particularly consistent in those who have a weight problem.

Having discovered when and why, I next had to determine how this pattern could be changed. Obviously, in view of decades of little or no success, we needed a powerful intervention, far-reaching and pervasive. This intervention needed to provide a strong framework for change in lifestyles in which food played a larger-than-desired part.

Over the years, I developed strategies to deal effectively with each of these antecedents. In order to change habits, people needed to structure food intake appropriately. They had to learn about nutrition and how to modify eating habits. I designed an extensive series of classes and workshops to meet these objectives.

It was much more complex to eliminate boredom. I had to analyze lifestyles to identify specific voids and unmet needs. Each individual had to discover activities other than eating which were rewarding and capable of fulfilling needs in their own personal search for a fulfilling lifestyle.

As I had expected, stress proved to be the most complex and involved antecedent to modify, often requiring major life changes. People reached amazing conclusions and made major decisions when they placed their own health and emotional happiness as a number one priority. I have seen people change careers, relationships, and geographical locations of their residence, as well as make very significant changes in handling day-to-day stresses and situations.

As time went on I recognized the need to refine the program. I was not satisfied with the institutional environment available to Duke. Also I could not effectively mold the positive, supportive atmosphere which I felt was necessary to foster a trusting open environment. It was at this juncture that I founded Structure House. Structure House has evolved into a program aimed at acquiring a healthy lifestyle by learning the behaviors associated with a healthy lifestyle. Of course, healthy lifestyles include proper cardiovascular fitness. Exercise has been one particularly important refinement directed toward reducing the health risks produced by a sedentary lifestyle which usually accompanies excess weight.

As time continues, I will make additional improvements. By making critical observations I will add to the process. In this way Structure House faithfully reflects the problem with which it works. Weight control is an ongoing process and as such is never finished.

I met Jimmy Coco in January of 1973 while still in the early stages of my work. We knew he was coming well ahead of time and naturally wondered how he would adjust to our clinic. We never provided a spa atmosphere and wondered whether he would be willing to work on the problem from our perspective. At the same time, we were concerned whether other patients would allow him, if he were serious, to attend to his own needs in peace.

The overall response was just short of being incredible. Jimmy was serious about his problem, came prepared to accept our approach, and proved to be down to earth. He made everyone around him feel particularly comfortable with his presence and everyone respected his need to be here. Over the years, after seeing Jimmy in many situations, I have learned that he has a remarkable ability to put people at ease and to give them a feeling that they truly are getting to know him, while at the same time being completely himself.

I had an immediate liking for this man and yet saw clearly the pain he was experiencing. He was approaching the age at which his mother had died and his continued obesity was proving to be both increasingly frightening and depressing.

In this way, Jimmy exhibited the essential prerequisite for anyone serious about undertaking weight loss and a quality we look for when our patients come to us. One must experience both a physical and psychological pain due to the excess weight to undertake this process effectively.

Jimmy appeared generally industrious in what he undertook. But he made a point of attending and participating in workshops and classes in his own way. At times, I wondered whether he was listening as seriously as I had hoped. It was difficult for Jimmy not to keep everyone laughing at times. I did not know whether he was just being himself or creating a defense. He kept his diary faithfully, learning how to use it in preparation for the time he was to go home. He attended *every* meal with the exception of those for which he did restaurant practice. His weight loss was exceptional and represents one of the most outstanding weight losses with us for a 30-day stay. He seemed to be showing the behavior which has proven critical for long-term results among our patients—an active participation in what we have to offer.

At the end of his stay, Jimmy was ready to go home. He had developed an attachment to us, even asking what we were going to do for entertainment now that he was leaving. I told him we had booked Dom DeLuise for the next two weeks. He said that was okay, and he would keep in touch anyway.

He did! In fact, he maintained particularly close contact, calling me frequently when he encountered difficulties. Jimmy was doing the next thing that successful patients have done. He realized that the process of weight control extended beyond his stay with us and the close contact was important as he continued to search for the antecedents to his unstructured eating. At times, I was concerned as to whether he was expecting too much from the treatment and not enough from himself.

As is so often the pattern with my patients, Jimmy's problems were in part rather direct and in part quite complex. Because of his ethnic background, habits played a large part in his overeating. Because of his show business lifestyle, stress played a very deep and involved role. Jimmy quite successfully was able to use what he learned to deal with the former. In part he made his ethnic background an asset and has learned to restructure his eating to maintain his food tradition while maintaining a good control over calories. Jimmy has developed many enjoyable and highly structured recipes over the years, some of which we now use at Structure House.

His sometimes chaotic lifestyle has been something else, however, and has always represented a challenge to structured eating. His continual encounter with certain sets of circumstances gradually proved to be depressing to Jimmy. This continued struggle preceded an important confrontation that took place shortly after Structure House was opened. As a result of this confrontation, I asked him to attend all our workshops and classes again. For one thing, I had added many new sessions and refined others since our early days. For another, I had wondered to what extent he had listened that first time in 1974. Jimmy soon realized we were not preaching a rigid philosophy for all to follow blindly. Jimmy had finally reached the conclusion that is essential for all our patients who succeed: Structure House is really a place where you learn a problem-solving approach, where you learn a way of *thinking* about and dealing with your weight problems. Though you learn a basic set of principles, you are able to apply these to your unique situation. In a sense, people take from us what is necessary to make weight control successful for them. Jimmy, having come to this point, now exhibits increased control over his eating. Yet, I believe he realizes that the job is never done. Weight control is a way of life and an ongoing process which each person can control if he chooses to.

Part I

How I Got This Way: The Whole Story

1. Fat Beginnings

I never had a weight problem until I was nine years old.

According to my older sister, Lucia, who mothered me from the day I was born, I was a poor eater as a child. No matter what I was served, I would pick at my food and stare at my plate. Strange as it may seem, *I* didn't even like pasta as a child! I just didn't like food. Period.

But Lucia was determined to have me grow up big, healthy, and strong, and she resorted to a bag of tricks to get me to eat. She was relentless, especially when she was trying to get me to eat vegetables which, like most kids, I hated. Undeterred, she would find ways of disguising them. When I wasn't looking, she would sneak a broccoli spear into a piece of rolled beef, stash a leaf of cooked escarole under a sliced meatball, or bury a handful of green peas in a mountain of mashed potatoes. (To this day, I don't like escarole.) Then, humming a vague tune, she would offer me her special concoction, hoping I would swallow the bait before catching on to her subterfuge. Other times, she would try coaxing me with promises of a new toy, a pony ride, or a trip to the park if I would just eat everything on my plate. Or she'd use diversionary tactics—like reading a story or playing a game—and wait for the opportune moment to strike. As I gaped at the mechanical wonder of a toy airplane whooshing through the air to cries of "Watch the airplane," she would slip in another morsel of food.

When I reflect on those early years, remembering the loves and hates, the ploys and tricks, the hidden resentments, the anger and frustrations, I realize that my sister and I were playing a winning game. Despite the deceptions and the pressures and the force-feeding, I learned a fundamental truth. Food is love.

Whenever we reminisce about childhood and the talk turns to what I looked like when I was a child, she always whips out a sepia-toned photograph of a thin seven-year-old in a skimpy bathing suit, posing on a rock. This is supposed to be me, and if you look long enough and hard enough, there *is* a faint resemblance. I stare at that skinny kid in the faded photograph, finally recognizing myself by the theatrical stance, and I realize that except for those first early years of my life, there never has been a time when I didn't have a weight problem.

I had a routine tonsillectomy when I was nine. I had been complaining about a sore throat. The diagnosis was "enlarged tonsils," the family doctor recommended that they be removed, and my parents arranged for the surgery. In those days, tonsillectomies were fashionable. At the first complaint of a sore throat, children were almost automatically packed off to a hospital for a "T-and-A," a tonsillectomy and adenoid operation. The adenoids were removed for good measure.

Today, physicians are of two minds about whether tonsillectomies are advisable. For a variety of reasons, many doctors feel that removing tonsils is not a good idea; that, for the most part, tonsillectomies are probably unnecessary; and that sore throats in children usually clear up without surgery, especially if treated with antibiotics. Today, doctors are more reluctant to remove glands and tissues whose function is not fully understood. Things might have been different if they had felt that way when I was a kid. Without that tonsillectomy, I might never have had a weight problem. Though I was terrified at first of surgery, my parents won me over by describing the ice cream feasts to come and pointing out that I would be in the hospital only overnight. They also promised me the latest comic books. Seduced and distracted by the promises of those goodies, I became less jittery. Visions of Breyer's hand-dipped ice cream danced in my head as I went under the anesthetic—vanilla, chocolate, strawberry, the three main flavors they made then. My last conscious thought was of chocolate. As promised, when I awoke after the operation, my mother was standing by with quarts of ice cream as well as the latest issues of Captain Marvel, Batman, and Superman. Barely able to speak above a hoarse whisper, I devoured the ice cream, even swapping flavors with other tonsillectomy patients in the children's ward. It was like an assembly line of flavors all moving down a conveyor belt. As I lapped up the remains of my third container of chocolate ice cream, a tonsillectomy seemed like fun. It was quick. It was easy. It was almost painless and I could gorge myself on gallons of ice cream without hearing a peep out of my sister. Once my friends heard about my burgeoning collection of comic books and my ice cream extravaganza, they were envious. There was a sudden epidemic of sore throats in the neighborhood and an increase in tonsillectomies. For a while there was a run on ice cream and comic books. Ice cream and comic books can be a powerful lure.

Sometime after the tonsillectomy—I don't remember exactly when—I became a fat kid almost overnight. For reasons that I did not understand, I was suddenly transformed from a bony, emaciated child to a round, chubby preadolescent. While it must have been a gradual transformation, it felt like a sudden metamorphosis. Later that same year, my weight suddenly shot up.

Puzzled by the abrupt change in my weight, I asked my parents why I had suddenly become so fat. "Don't worry. It's nothing. It'll go away. You'll see. It's from the operation." At the time, unconscious of the complex physiological and psychological causes for the dramatic change in my weight, I bought the story that the tonsillectomy caused the physical change, believing that my parents were right and that, in time, I would become my old self again. At ten, I was very trusting. I don't think I ever got a satisfactory answer to my questions. But, frankly, I don't think my parents knew the answers. My sister is still convinced that if it hadn't been for the routine tonsillectomy, I would never have had a lifelong weight problem. Today, I don't buy that. At first, being chubby didn't bother me—not at age ten—except for my clothes. They were so snug, I felt as if I were back in swaddling clothes. My mother, who was occasionally em-

ployed as a finisher in the garment industry and who was
experienced at sewing, was always snipping and patching
and tacking and gluing. Buttons popped. Seams split. Zippers broke. With her experienced hand she was always
there when the crisis occurred. Later we bought my clothes
in fat men's shops. I hated that. I wasn't just growing like
most kids. I was growing in several different directions. My
thighs were so heavy they rubbed against each other when I
walked, wearing out my pants. So my mother would rein-
force them with heavy patches of mismatched material.
Whenever I caught anybody staring at my mother's handiwork,
I could feel my face getting hot, and I knew I was turning
red.

In those days, most kids pressed to answer that silly,
tiresome question, "What do you want to be when you grow
up?" almost always answered, "I want to be a fireman"or "I
want to be a baseball player." But by then I was already
dreaming another dream. I knew I wanted to be an actor.
And after seeing Charles Laughton and Paul Muni and all the
other wonderful character actors, I knew that being an actor
did not mean having to be a gymnast. My goals were
different. So while my friends ran through the routines like
Olympic champs, I often just sat on the sidelines, admiring
them and complimenting them on their physical dexterity,
kidding around all the while about why I couldn't join in.
Also, I wasn't going to stick my neck out and embarrass
myself by attempting physical feats I knew I couldn't pull off.

Though I was actually born in Manhattan on 177th Street
and St. Nicholas Avenue in Washington Heights, I grew up
in the Bronx. My Sicilian father, after first emigrating to
Argentina and remaining long enough to marry my mother
and begin raising a family, settled in America. Like thousands of other peasant farmers and unskilled laborers from
southern Italy who came looking for "bread and work," my
parents settled in one of New York's immigrant neighborhoods.

Growing up Italian meant having a backyard fig tree.
Growing up Italian meant making homemade wine. Growing
up Italian meant raising homegrown parsley and basil and
luscious tomatoes in a window-box garden. And growing up
Italian meant being raised on antiquated, old-world ideas
about social and sexual mores. For years, my poor sister

was not allowed to wear lipstick or high-heeled shoes. If my parents had had their way, they would have permanently kept her in black mourning dress under the watchful eye of an elderly duenna. Still, when the time was right, she fell in love, had a traditional wedding and raised a lovely third-generation family. With all the ethnic dilemmas, the upheavals of old world and new, the lingering poverty, growing up Italian meant growing up with a lot of tradition, a lot of love and a lot of pasta.

As in Italy, breakfast was never a big deal. For breakfast, I usually had a half a loaf of Italian bread, buttered heavily and dunked into my coffee. But it could just as easily have been a soggy leftover cannoli, a thick slice of chocolate cake, or even cold leftover spaghetti. My mother used to prepare a peasant dish that was made with hard stale bread, soaked in water, dipped in olive oil, seasoned with pepper, and baked. It was so lowly, it didn't even have a name. If I had to give a name to that dish today, I would call it "la miseria." Loosely translated, "la miseria" means poverty, southern Italian style. This lowly meal of hard pieces of Italian bread kept those starving peasants alive. Although it was not a usual breakfast food, that commonplace "miseria" meal was one of my favorite breakfast treats. The attractive magazine ads for Kellogg's Corn Flakes or Jack Armstrong's catchy jingle for Wheaties, "the breakfast of champions," never altered our family eating habits. We hummed ditties along with all the other "All-American Boys," but we never rushed out to buy the cereals. Our breakfasts were strictly ethnic.

Later, when I needed information for a passport, I learned that my mother had actually been born in Argentina. I assumed that my Argentine-born mother was Spanish; in fact, her father was Italian and her mother was Spanish. It's a hybrid family tree. So it was a revelation when I was almost in my mid-twenties: I was one-quarter Spanish—there was a strain of Castilian blood in our Italian veins. I pushed hard for that Spanish connection! Somehow it made us different. Still, we were brought up Italian.

We lived on the ground floor of a small walk-up at 2820 Middletown Road in the Bronx. The number 2820 adds up to 12, a number that has *always* figured in my life. I was born on March 21. My collaborator, Marion, was born on March 12. The publication date of this book is February 1 (2/1). Spooky. I see signs in things.

Though our apartment was small for a family of five, it looked enormous to my child's eyes. My parents had the only real bedroom. At night, with portable roll-out beds, the dining room became a bedroom for my brother and me. My sister's bedroom doubled as a family room. My brother, Frankie, used to practice the piano there, while my sister, growing through adolescence, congregated with her teenage friends there. Everything that was meaningful to me until I was seventeen happened in that apartment on Middletown Road.

My mother died of a cerebral hemorrhage there. She had never been ill, but she suddenly developed phlebitis and within weeks died of an embolism. As there was no effective treatment for phlebitis then, the doctor suspected she would die, although he did not share this information with the family. Because the family was unaware of the critical nature of her illness, her death was quite a shock. That same year, my newly married sister moved into the apartment with her husband. My older brother, Frankie, an entertainer who played the accordion, left for war from there. My widowed father, visiting his native Italy several years after my mother died, brought home a new Italian bride.

And at seventeen, living at home with my father and stepmother, I landed my first job in the theater with a touring company. From then on, I was on my own. Later, when I visited my childhood home, the apartment was much smaller than my memory had painted it. I felt as though I were in a shoe box.

I made my theatrical debut at seventeen in the title role of King Cole with the Clare Tree Major Children's Theater. My salary was forty dollars a week. Traveling cross-country, hauling scenery in a big red truck, we played school auditoriums to audiences of screaming kids. Children can be difficult both on and off stage.

As the company's fat character actor, I got to play all the splashy parts, gargantuan potentates, and portly kings, bejeweled and bedecked in flashy costumes. The great Kublai

Khan, the emperor and founder of the Mongol dynasty in medieval China, was my favorite role.

I was not only the company character actor, but also the company manager, an official title that entailed various administrative duties. I had to make sure the actors were paid on time, keep track of booking schedules, and get us from one town to another in time for performances. Having to get from places like San Antonio, Texas, to Fort Worth, Texas, in the same day was long and arduous. We put in very long hours.

While officially I was actor-manager for the company, unofficially I became the company cook. With very little money, we stayed at the cheapest hotels and ate meagerly, often preparing hotplate meals in our hotel rooms, violating well-known fire regulations. Despite the hotel regulations against home-cooking, we always smuggled in a hotplate, ignoring the signs: *No Cooking Allowed.* The company was always impressed with my ability to whip up an Italian meal. For years, we dined on spaghetti and meatballs.

After three years with the Clare Tree Major Children's Theater, I was ready for the big time. I thought. The big time was a summer stock job in a small New England paper mill town. Although I don't remember the name of the town anymore, I do remember the logs floating down the river and the ever-present smell of paper in the air.

In the big time, we worked for room and board which is to say there was very little room and practically no board. The company lived community style in a loft over the theater. Reminiscent of the famous scene in *It Happened One Night* in which Clark Gable and Claudette Colbert are separated by a blanket and a clothesline, the loft was partitioned off with sheets. The girls lived on one side, the boys on the other. We slept on old army cots.

We worked long hours during the day building and painting scenery and getting it on stage so we would have a set to work in at night. Despite the hard work, it was worth it when we heard the applause.

And in addition to everything else we did, we had to prepare our own meals. Food was rationed, so the refrigerator was kept under lock and key. There was no way of getting at the food after the evening performance.

That summer not only did I begin my professional career as a fat character actor, but I also began building a reputation as a fat character actor with a flair for cooking. Cooking has always been a happy pastime for me. I enjoy cooking. I learned it at my mother's apron strings. That summer and - for many more summers to come, we dined luxuriously on sweat, dreams and spaghetti and meatballs. I was good at all three.

One day, as I made television rounds and sat in a waiting room jammed with other twenty-year-old aspirants, it suddenly occurred to me as I looked around that everybody was beautiful. The room was full of beautiful people. There was no one there who looked like me. There were no twenty-year-olds with bulging thighs waiting to audition. I felt like an outcast. Like a misfit. Like I didn't belong. Suddenly I thought, "Fat is not beautiful. It's not true what my mother told me. It was a lie. I'm not special because I'm fat. I'm ugly. They lied to me." As I sat there, waiting for my interview, I could feel everybody staring at me. Who did they think I was? Certainly not an actor. The telephone repair man? The maintenance man? "How can I compete with these beautiful people?" I thought. "What chance do I have? What chance does a fat, ugly person like me have against these beautiful people?" For the first time in my life, I became aware of being fat. I became self-conscious. I didn't like being fat anymore. I didn't like the way I looked. I wanted to look like them. I wanted to look like the other people in that room. I didn't want to look like an ugly old man at twenty. I didn't get the job that afternoon.

Though I was probably always bothered by the weight, I finally admitted it to myself without knowing what to do about it.

2. Confessions of a Diet Junkie

In those days, I knew nothing about nutrition or about dieting, since I came from a nondieting background. I began to try to diet on my own. I ate the same foods, trying to cut back. But cutting back simply didn't make a dent in my weight. It stayed way up there and I stayed fat and uncomfortable.

And while I was trying to climb the broken ladder of success, my weight and my career were at a standstill. In television commercials, it was the time of non-ethnics. Sponsors didn't want dark, swarthy Italians selling their snowy white detergents. It took a helluva long time before I landed my job as "Willie the Plumber," on a Drano commercial. After considerable persistence by casting director Maxime Marx, the daughter of Groucho Marx, I finally became "Willie the Plumber." My father, who was still alive at the time, was very proud, boasting to his Italian neighbors, "Do you know my son is a television plumber?" For me, Willie meant I could eat.

I was 250 pounds for a long time. Until *Auntie Mame*. When I was cast in Constance Bennett's road company of *Auntie Mame*, I felt as if I had arrived. To me, Miss Bennett was big time. By then, I was a member of Actors' Equity, the actors' union, which meant I could earn a little more money, and I felt up again. When I began working again, I almost forgot about my weight problem.

One night, while I was in Miss Bennett's dressing room, just before show time, she turned to me and said what all fat people hear, "You have such a wonderful face. You really should lose some weight. And, darling, it isn't healthy at your age." Moved by her concern, I vowed in Constance Bennett's dressing room to finally lick the damn weight problem. I was going to do it. My pal in that company was another fat actor, Roger Carmel.

"Roger, we're going on a diet. We are going to lose weight. I don't know how. But we're going to diet. I promised Constance Bennett we would." "What do you mean?" he said. "I don't know how to diet. I've never dieted." "That's the trouble," I said. "That's why you're fat. That's why I'm fat. We've got to start now. We're young. We're just starting out. This is the time to do it. We'll find a way. We'll ask around. We'll talk to people. We'll find the answer. It can't be that hard. Just think (I said), we'll be on the road for nine months. If we lost ten pounds a month, by the time we get back we'll have lost ninety pounds. We'll be sensational. We'll be the talk of the town. That alone is worth it. Nobody will recognize us." "Yeah," he said, momentarily frightened. "I don't want that. We want people to recognize us, don't we? We want to be recognizable types, don't we?" "Can't we be thin and still be recognizable types?" I asked. "I mean, I still want to work in the theater." I said, "Well, sure—of course we do. Of course, we will. But just think of the shock, the surprise. At first, they'll be shocked. But once they recover, they'll recognize us again."

So Roger and I put our heads together and devised a diet plan. It was a potpourri of bits and pieces of information that we had picked up out of the air practically. We starved all day, cut out snacks, sweets, breads, and cakes, and in the evening had an enormous dinner of fish, eggs, or meat. For breakfast we had half a grapefruit and black coffee.

In nine months, I lost one hundred pounds. So did Roger. But I also felt woozy from starving. It affected my concentration onstage. I suppose, emotionally, since I was starving, I was obsessed with that one big evening meal of the day. Unaware that the diet was totally unbalanced because the weight loss was so spectacular, we thought it was a winner. Later, I learned that except for the protein it lacked all other essential nutrients.

As the weight was coming off, I even thought Miss Bennett was making goo-goo eyes at me. I've always had a vivid imagination. For me, it was a diet "first." Being thin for the first time ever was a startling experience. I couldn't wait to get back home for everybody to see me. Without realizing it, too, I had incorporated the buddy system. For me, the buddy system is an important adjunct to the success of any diet. It's always easier *with* someone.

With his new trim figure, Roger became a peacock. Convinced he was now a double for Tyrone Power and absolutely irresistible to women, he made a pass at every maid, extra, cleaning woman, and actress in the company. He became the town stud, the Burt Reynolds of that era.

When I got home there were shrieks and screams and almost hysteria. My sister thought I was suffering from an incurable disease. Friends screamed, "Oh no, what have you done?" "Too much, too much." "You look sick." "Are you dying?" "What's the matter?" "You went too far." Despite the panic, they were happy too. They knew how much it meant to me to have lost that much weight. I had a tremendous feeling of satisfaction, of elation, for the first time in my life. I filled the apartment with mirrors. I pranced naked in front of them, admiring myself from every angle. My God, I thought, this is me. James Coco, former fat actor. I was shocked myself at the way I looked. Roger was right. I didn't recognize myself. Who the hell else would recognize us? Maybe we'd never work again—as Roger was afraid might happen. I didn't care. So I'd never work again. I was thin. Roger was ecstatic too. This was the first time since I was ten that I was thin. This was the first time since that tonsillectomy. I threw out all my fat clothes. Bought a whole new wardrobe. I went from a size 48 to a size 32 pants. In my new duds, I paraded around town. I wanted the world to see that James Coco, the formerly fat actor, was now a thin character actor. I almost took an ad in *Variety*, the industry's trade paper, to announce that I was ready to play any thin character part available. No more fat character parts. I was sick of them. I didn't have enough money so I didn't take out the ad. At that time, it cost approximately five hundred dollars for a full-page ad. Thank God I didn't, because *within six months, I had regained the weight.* This time I wanted to hide my head in the sand,

write to my congressman for a change of address, move out
to the desert with the iguanas. They wouldn't recognize me.
What would my sister say now? What would my friends say?
I kept thinking, when are they going to finally notice? I
actually got some people saying, "You know, you look much
better. You look like your old self again." When I started to
get *that* old routine, I thought, "Ugh, I'm done for. I'm back
to square one." I didn't try dieting like that again for several
years—not until I went out on the road with *Shot in the
Dark*. I decided to give it another try. Maybe this time it
would work. Maybe this time I would find the magic formula
that would keep it off. For the second time I went on the
diet that we had pieced together from scraps of information—
starving all day, eating only at night—and crying myself to
sleep. History repeated itself. After nine months, I had lost
another 100 pounds. Coming home, I made a second thin
man entrance. Everybody reacted the same way. I scared
my sister, floored the neighbors, startled my friends. I
threw out all my old fat clothes. Bought a whole new
wardrobe, and thought about taking out an ad in *Variety*.
Guess what happened? Six months later I had regained all
the weight. I was back up to size 48 all over again.

After the sorry failures of those two spectacular attempts
at losing weight on my own, I was discouraged and depressed,
convinced I'd never make it. I was locked into a pattern of
dieting that went up and down and up and down like a ride
on a Coney Island roller coaster. "It's no use. I'm doomed,"
I decided. "I'm a loser." Twice I lost 100 pounds, and both
times I gained it all back. Something inside my wounded,
frustrated, angry, humiliated psyche wanted me to keep
trying until I won. Everybody loves a winner. At that time,
secretly, I suppose, I still longed for a Robert Taylor
silhouette— the trim waistline, the long, taut legs—along
with the chiseled features. In short, I wanted that strikingly
handsome Taylor look which was fixed in my memory—his
intent gaze at the fabulous Garbo playing his beloved Camille.
I even envied his black, shiny, wavy hair (mine was already
beginning to go). Being a sentimental realist, I knew it
wasn't too likely I could look like Robert Taylor, but at
thirty I could still dream.

In 1964 almost on the heels of *A Shot in the Dark*, I got

my first big movie break, a bit part in *Ensign Pulver,* a comedy sequel to *Mister Roberts,* about the unsung heroes of the navy of World War II. It was shot in Acapulco, Mexico.

One of the worst films ever made, *Ensign Pulver* crops up regularly on the late late show like a bad dream. Featured as the young ensign was Robert Walker, Jr., the son of Jennifer Jones and the late Robert Walker. Other bit players were Jack Nicholson, Larry (J.R. on *Dallas*) Hagman, and Peter Marshall, the M. C. of "Hollywood Squares." Heading the cast were Burl Ives as the martinet captain and Walter Matthau as the weary understanding doctor. I can only tell you that the whole experience was a bomb.

I bumped into Jack Nicholson one night at Alfredo's Trattoria, a popular Italian restaurant in Greenwich Village. "Will you ever forget *Ensign Pulver,*" he asked. "Never," I answered. On "Hollywood Squares," Peter Marshall commented, "Remember *Ensign Pulver?*" "Yes," I nodded. Some things are hard to forget.

On a diet of Mexican enchiladas, tacos, tortillas, refried beans, and black bean sandwiches—delivered to the ship which was anchored in the middle of the Pacific—the inevitable happened.

I was back to looking like a character actor by the end of the film, having piled on another 25 pounds. I almost looked like a juvenile as the cameras began to roll.

As I floundered in search of a permanent cure or an alchemist's magic or a scientific breakthrough that would save me from this incurable disease, I started on my dietmania and drugs. Success did *not* feel like it was just around the corner.

In the 1950s and 1960s, everybody was popping diet pills. I was still taking them in the 1970s. Without actually knowing what we were taking, we were popping white round tablets, or orange-colored pills, or dark brown time-release capsules. They were anorexiants or appetite suppressants. Part stimulant, they are often called pep pills. On the black market today they are called "uppers," or "speed," but to ordinary mortals like me, they were just diet pills. Because they seemed to work so effectively we gobbled them up like so many penny candies. Only later did many of us learn that those colorful, innocuous-looking pills that came in a variety of shapes and colors and sizes and that gave us such a terrific lift were amphetamines, a dangerous habit-forming drug. At the time, they were just a simple, straightforward, easy-to-get diet pill. All you had to do was go to your doctor, weigh in, pay your money, and he would give you that envelope of precious pills. They were effective. They killed my appetite for a time. I lost weight. They made me feel good. I was happy. High on diet pills, I was overstimulated physically, bustling about my apartment looking for an outlet for that excess energy. Although no great fan of housework, I can honestly boast that during the diet pill craze, I had the cleanest apartment on the block. I was always on my hands and knees, scrubbing, polishing, vacuuming, and cleaning, rubbing down the bathroom tile to a soft patina, waxing the kitchen floor, or polishing the mirrors in my foyer until they sparkled like the Hall of Mirrors at the Palace of Versailles. Straight through the night, I would work at the kitchen table, feverishly polishing the silver, sorting out the flatware until each individual piece was safely back in its felt pocket. Or I would shampoo my Edward Fields cream-colored rug (always a problem color), trying hopelessly to get rid of the cigarette marks that a friend (or I) always managed to make in the most conspicuous corner. And although washing windows has never been my favorite chore, I washed every tiny little windowpane, perched precariously on a short stepladder that never comfortably reaches the top window, risking life and limb since I lived on the eleventh floor. Several times I almost wrenched my back, lugging a heavy potted palm across the floor. And when I ran out of things to do, I would start all over again. "How did I miss that spot on that knife?" I thought. Physically exhausted, I worked until the amphetamines wore off. Sometimes, still unable to sleep but having run out of work, I would sit in my black leather chair, staring into space, listening to the night sounds—a pair of late night revelers, homeward bound, harmonizing "Sweet Adeline," off-key, or the screaming of fire engines—and then I would catch the morning light.

While I was losing weight on the amphetamines, I quickly acquired a tolerance for them and had to increase the daily dosage. Although I started out by taking one a day, I gradually increased the number first to two a day and then to three, then to four, until finally I stopped counting. I was no longer taking them to kill my appetite; now I wanted them for that high. Instead of starting the day with a morning cigarette, I started with a little white pill and a glass of water. I couldn't get through the day without my pills. Since I was also taking sleeping pills for insomnia, I was on "uppers" by day and "downers" by night, feeling simultaneously elated and depressed, fluctuating between high and low moods. I was going through Jekyll-and-Hyde personality swings: affectionate one minute and raging the next. I was irritable and jumpy, snapping at my friends. Without knowing amphetamines were addictive, I got hooked on speed.

Even my closest friends who have never failed me stopped calling. I was too much to handle. I must have been a monster during that period. The personality change was so schizoid, none of my friends wanted to deal with me anymore. My behavior became too bizarre and unpredictable.

One day I read an article in *New York* magazine about the dangers of amphetamines. It was an eye-opener. After reading about what happens to amphetamine addicts—how desperate they become for that daily fix, the suicide attempts, the psychotic episodes, the changes in personality, the dependency and mainlining (taking amphetamine by injection)—I vowed to kick the habit.

Late in November, when everybody was out of town visiting friends and families and getting ready for Thanksgiving dinners, I woke up feeling groggy from the sleeping pill I took the night before. When I reached for my first fix of the day, there were no pills. Panicky, I ransacked the apartment, taking everything apart, but there were no pills anywhere. On a long holiday weekend, I had no pills, no prescription, and no doctor. Suddenly I thought: I can't go to my sister's for Thanksgiving dinner in this condition. She'll know. To keep her from finding out that I was a speed freak, I canceled Thanksgiving dinner. I didn't care about Thanksgiving or the holidays or anything. That weekend, without realizing what was happening, I went "cold turkey." Because there was no way I could get a fix, I was forced into a cure. I went to bed late Friday night and slept for fourteen hours—the first time I had ever done that in my life. When I woke up, I was exhausted but I knew I would never go back to pills again. By the end of the long weekend, I was beginning to feel more like myself again. Living on pills, going without sleep, being "hopped up" all the time is not the answer. Being a junkie is not the answer. It's a horrible way. It's a frightening road to take. Thank God, amphetamines are harder to get these days.

It was about that time that Dr. Herman Taller, a Brooklyn obstetrician and gynecologist, wrote his controversial book, *Calories Don't Count.* Without completely understanding Dr. Taller's theory of weight reduction, I jumped on the Taller bandwagon. Only after years of experience, when I was sharper and more sophisticated about diets, did I realize that *Calories Don't Count* was just another high-fat diet with a catchy title and a twist. The gimmick, of course, was polyunsaturated fats—the fats associated with low cholesterol—but many people, misinterpreting the title, believed that by eating polyunsaturated fats they could eat all the foods they wanted and still lose weight. That's what I thought too.

Taller, whose underlying message was "Eat fat and get thin" or "Fat melts away fat," recommended taking two tablespoons of polyunsaturated oils before each meal—either safflower or corn oil. He preferred safflower. That always made me gag. His theory was that there was a chemical fat imbalance in overweight people that prevented the proper release of stored-up fat. Polyunsaturated fats would restore the balance, he claimed, setting up a chain reaction that would break down those fatty deposits. "To lose fat," Dr. Taller wrote, "you must make your body consume its stored fat." By eating fats, he went on, "you set in motion a process which stimulates the pituitary gland and gets this fat-burning going at a higher rate. The obese person not only burns the fat he eats; his system gets so fired up that it burns the fat he has accumulated over the years." By eating polyunsaturated fats, "you set in motion a happy cycle. You stimulate body production of certain hormones which work to release fats stored around the body." Scientific gobbledygook that two million dieters—who bought his book and hung on every word, hoping for a get-thin-quick scheme—swallowed whole. I did, too. I stocked up on polyunsaturated oil, drowned my food in it, saturated my salads with it, took it straight when I didn't retch. And later, when CDC (Calories Don't Count) safflower oil capsules hit the market, I swallowed them like so many jelly beans.

Despite Taller's claim that "fat melts fat," in my case, "fat begat fat." I gained, and as for Dr. Taller—he almost went to jail. In 1962, after seizing *Calories Don't Count* as a fraud, the government indicted Dr. Taller on charges of mail fraud, conspiracy, and violation of food and drug regulations. In an apparent tie-in with Cove Vitamins and Pharmaceuticals, Inc., a drug company marketing the capsules, Taller was accused of promoting the sale of his book by the sale of the capsules. He was found guilty, accused of foisting a worthless scheme on a gullible public, fined $7,000 and placed on two years' probation. In his own defense, Taller—who had struggled all his life with fat—testified that he was living proof of the efficacy of his theory. In twelve years, he said, he had lost 104 pounds, slimming down to 171 pounds. Had I known that it had taken Dr. Taller twelve years to lose 104 pounds, I would have burned the book. I understand it's a collector's item. To his credit, he did make the public aware of polyunsaturated fats.

Dieting became a way of life for me. I tried every new diet that came along, however bizarre, kooky, mixed-up, obvious, or crooked. The results were always the same. I would lose and gain and lose and gain, plateauing-out on some diets, gaining on others. Once I got on that diet treadmill, it took a lifetime to get off. Whatever anybody was selling, I bought—like the bananas and cream diet. How is anybody going to lose weight on a diet of bananas and cream? It was somebody's aberration and I fell for it. Actually, the bananas and cream diet is a one-food idea of dieting that crops up periodically. Someone who eats unlimited quantities of only one food will lose weight, so the theory goes. It's silly. Yet, when I was doing *Such Good Friends,* I remember seeing Dyan Cannon eating grapes. All day she ate nothing but grapes, which she carried around the studio in a brown paper bag. That was a one-food diet idea, too, I think. Well, Dyan is so terrific-looking, I find it hard to believe that grapes had anything to do with Dyan Cannon's sensational figure. Maybe she just liked grapes.

When I tried Dr. Irwin Maxwell Stillman's *The Doctor's*

Quick Weight Loss Diet, nicknamed the water diet, I ran into a big problem. That doctor ordered: drink at least eight glasses of water a day. And that was in addition to all the coffee, tea, and diet sodas I normally consumed in a day. Since I was always gung-ho at first with any new diet, I put up a chart on my kitchen bulletin board, neatly divided into five columns: water, coffee, diet soda, tea, and "other," as a reminder of what I was drinking. In the best of all possible worlds, I suppose, the column marked "other" would have been reserved for alcohol. On the Stillman high-protein, zero-carbohydrate, low-fat diet, alcohol was prohibited because in the digestive process it changes to glycogen, a form of carbohydrate. At first, it worked fine. The columns were neat and clean. The lines were straight. The check marks were distinct. And I knew exactly how much "other" I was consuming. Then it all went down the drain. I made mistakes. I would tick off the wrong columns, checking coffee when I meant water, marking tea—which I hate—when I meant coffee. Heaven knows what I put under "other." Waterlogged, I felt as if I were floating out to sea. On that diet I had to know where every clean bathroom was from 14th Street to 55th Street. After drinking eight glasses of water a day, I could get the call at any given moment.

I met Dr. Stillman on the talk-show circuit once in Philadelphia when I was cohosting "The Mike Douglas Show" and another time in Burbank when I was appearing on the Johnny Carson show. An energetic, lively, wiry man in his early seventies, with a wonderful sense of humor, Dr. Stillman still had the same youthful physique that he had had as a student attending Bushwick High School in Brooklyn. He told us he had never had a weight problem. For some reason that bothered me—envy maybe, or doubts about the efficacy of his theories, or probably just a silly notion that not having suffered the agonies of being fat, he should not prescribe for the obese.

As we talked diets on the Douglas show, Dr. Stillman suddenly grabbed me by the ankle. "Yes," he said, "you have water retention." "How is drinking eight gallons of water a day going to help my water retention?" I answered. "Not eight gallons," he said, "eight glasses." "Oh." "It'll flush it out," he said. "Oh. Drinking eight glasses of water will flush out the water?" I must be slow, I thought. Anyway, Dr. Stillman, having seen me prepare my ricotta–meatloaf dish on an earlier show, asked me for the recipe for his new diet book. Even in his new book, he was still pushing water. As my late dear friend, Totie Fields, said to him, "Jesus Christ, I had to wear Pampers." I have often thought that because Stillman's was a gimmick diet, whenever I hadn't consumed the obligatory eight glasses of water a day, psychologically I thought I had blown the diet. I found myself going off. Gimmick diets do that to you. If you don't stick to it to the letter, you feel as if you've blown it.

In fairness, there was a method to Dr. Stillman's madness. For complicated medical reasons, which I barely understood at the time, but which I accepted on faith, Dr. Stillman believed drinking plenty of fluids would prevent ketosis, an accumulation of excessive amounts of ketones. Ketones are a natural consequence of carbohydrate deficiency. In the complex process of burning fat, ketones are produced and, if not completely burned, build up in the blood and urine, creating the condition of ketosis which in turn can cause gout in people who are susceptible to that, and other kidney-related complications. Drinking fluids would flush out the ketones from the body. Whether it flushed out mine, I'll never know.

On Dr. Robert C. Atkins' *Dr. Atkins' Diet Revolution,* a high-fat, low-carbohydrate diet, I had a different problem: the high fat. After about a week of stuffing myself on Atkins foods—bacon cheeseburgers, lobster with butter sauce, bacon and eggs, eggs Benedict with hollandaise, steak with bearnaise sauce—I developed an ugly, greasy taste in my mouth that I couldn't shake. It stuck to the roof of my mouth like rendered fat sitting in an old Crisco can on the kitchen window. From eating all that fat, I began to feel sick and nauseated and faint. At first, I suppose, the idea of being able to gorge myself—"eat as much as you want"—on those forbidden foods was titillating, but when my cholesterol levels and blood pressure shot all the way up, I backed off and decided to take another look. Unlike Taller, who practically invented polyunsaturated fats, Atkins went the other way. He passionately promoted foods high in saturated fats and cholesterol, which I had been told were risk factors for cardiovascular diseases. I couldn't take that chance. Not with my history. Carbohydrates, not fat, were the killer, according to Dr. Atkins. Get rid of carbohydrates, he declaimed, and it would be a whole new world. He said, "On a high-fat, low-carbohydrate diet, the body will have no carbohydrates to burn as fuel; therefore, it will mobilize fat from the soft, hanging, unsightly adipose tissues under the skin." Sounds terrific. It just didn't work with me.

In a doctor's office on New York's Upper East Side, a physician in a typical crisp white doctor's coat—I've blocked the name—was peddling the urine of pregnant women as a treatment for obesity. This gimmick was the brainchild of one Dr. Albert T.W. Simeons, who in the mid-1930s had treated young boys with Fröhlich's syndrome—the accumulation of fat around the hips, buttocks, and thighs that made boys look like girls. For a while, the accepted treatment for this syndrome was HCG, human chorionic gonadotropin, a growth hormone extracted from the urine of pregnant women.

Basing his work on experiments with Fröhlich patients, Simeons concocted a theory of weight reduction that combined HCG and the 500-calorie diet which he was already using with patients. Pretty soon, cashing in on the Simeons method, HCG fat clinics sprang up everywhere. At one time in California alone there were 80 weight-reduction medical clinics pushing the Simeons method.

Like most dieters looking for a quick fix, I decided to take a shot of HCG therapy. "I'll eat mud if it works," I told myself. That's how I came to be in a crowded waiting room furnished in Danish modern, waiting, along with other obese hopefuls, for my first urine injection. I felt like Ponce de Leon in search of the fountain of youth, but I wasn't so sure when I glanced at the 300-calorie diet that was distributed as part of the program. This was a slimmed-down version of the original Simeons diet—already pretty sparse at 500 calories. When you're on 300 calories a day, you measure food in eyedropper proportions. Breakfast was black coffee. Lunch was black coffee. Dinner was 3½ ounces of fish or chicken.

After giving me the first shot, the doctor disappeared. I never saw him again, but the injections continued, given each week by one of a team of harried nurses. Harried though they were, they managed to insert the needle in a different spot each week. The result was a checkerboard pattern of pinpricks. Beguiled by the lure of a magic cure, I kept swallowing the bait, waiting for the pregnant urine to melt away the fat—and forgetting for the moment that anyone on a 300-calorie diet will lose weight, no matter what is being injected. But when I began to feel like a pin cushion, I knew it was time to scout around for another diet. Besides, I was starving to death. Although in 1976 the Food and Drug Administration declared HCG ineffective, and warned Simeons-style clinics against making false claims, there still are diet hucksters selling the urine of pregnant women as a treatment for obesity.

Jerry Stiller called me one day, all excited about a diet he was on. (Jerry Stiller and Anne Meara are long-time friends.) "Listen," he said. "I want to tell you about this diet." "OK," I said. "Go ahead." "It's a water diet," he said, his voice husky with emotion. "A what?" I yelped. "It's a water diet," he repeated. "You just drink water." "Yes?" "Well, that's it." "What do you mean that's it? You mean that's all there is to it?" "No, no," he said, still sounding as if he were in seventh heaven. "You go to this place in the country. It's beautiful. There are a lot of trees there and you drink water. And they give you vitamin supplements too." Then I said, "You go away and drink water and get vitamin supplements. Well, it must be a very cheap diet. How much does it cost, Jerry?" When he told me I almost keeled over. "You mean, you actually go to a place where you drink water and get vitamin supplements and you pay that amount of money for it? Why don't you try it in your own apartment?" I asked. "It's not the same," he said. "Jerry," I said, "thanks for the call, but I think I'll pass. Is Anne there?" I don't know whether he heard me or not because he hung up. I didn't see any point in going someplace to pay for something you can get out of your own faucet. What Jerry was talking about, of course, was total fasting. Who needs it? And who needs a modified-fasting protein-sparing diet.

The last chance I didn't want was Robert Linn's *The Last Chance Diet*. It was too risky and in the long run just didn't pay off. I know actors who have developed serious complications from being on a liquid protein diet such as Dr. Linn's.

Doris Roberts, who costarred with me in *The Last of the Red Hot Lovers*, lost almost all her hair from Opti-Fast, a liquid protein product from Minnesota. And there was Charles Durning, that marvelous actor, with a chronic weight problem like mine. When I bumped into him one day at the Los Angeles airport, I had to turn back twice. I hardly recognized him because he had slimmed way down. He looked half his former size. "Charlie!" I screamed. "Hey," he shouted back, chuckling loudly. "You look terrific," I said. "I found it," he said. Puzzled for a minute, I said, "What? What did you find?" "The answer," he said. "The answer." "What answer?" I asked, as we tried to talk over the screaming sounds of the jets streaking across the California skies. Charlie said, "I finally found a diet that works for me." "How did you do it?" I asked, grabbing him by the arm as he flung his trenchcoat over his shoulder—or, am I thinking about a gesture he did with his characterization in *Queen of the Stardust Ballroom*, the award-winning television play with Maureen Stapleton? "Liquid protein," he uttered with the fervor of a religious convert. "I don't need food anymore," he said. "I don't even think about food. I have even forgotten what it feels like to chew." (Oops, I thought to myself. Trouble—remembering about Doris Roberts losing her hair.) Having learned a little bit about liquid protein diets, I sort of knew what to expect. But he was so enthusiastic about it, I didn't have the heart to tell about my doubts. The next time I saw Charlie, he had gained weight again. I didn't bring it up. Instead, I told him how wonderful I thought he was in *True Confessions*, which I had just seen. But then again, Charles Durning is wonderful in everything he does.

Believe it or not, there are people who actually have their jaws wired to lose weight. However desperate I may be, I balk at that kind of bizarre behavior. And even though I have a crackerjack oral surgeon like Dr. Stephen F. Goodman, I would never have my jaws wired. It certainly wouldn't improve my looks. Since I couldn't appear on stage or on television or on an interview show with chicken wire in my mouth, I would have to go into seclusion, like a bear hibernating, living off its fat. What if I landed a toothpaste commercial? What would I do then? Besides, even if my jaws were clamped shut with eighteen gauge steel, I would find a way of getting at the food. Using my Cuisinart, I could always puree a pizza and slurp it up with a straw.

I understand that this particular fad started in England. Obviously at her wits' end, a woman weighing 238 pounds had her mouth sealed by having a silver splint cemented to her teeth. (In the United States, the jaws are usually wired by placing a thin metal bar across the upper teeth, placing another bar across the lower teeth and running wire tightly between the two bars, preventing the jaws from opening.) With that silver splint in her mouth for months and on a liquid diet, the woman from England naturally lost weight. When the splint was finally removed she said, "I would smile if I could, but it hurts too much." I bet it did.

The Sleep Diet is another diet I rejected. On that one, a person is rendered almost comatose and fed intravenously for six months. As an insomniac I probably wouldn't go under anyway. Being out would make me very uneasy. I would worry about all the calls I'd miss. What if I were offered a new series, or a new film or a new play? No, sleeping is out. Dieting isn't easy.

I once seriously considered having a bypass, an intestinal operation for heavy weight reduction. For the extremely obese, it sounded like a medical breakthrough. I had heard that people with intractable obesity, hearing about this radical new treatment, flocked in droves for the operation. There were rumors that bypass patients had lost a hundred pounds in a hundred days. For them, dieting was obsolete. With a bypass, they could eat and gorge and binge and not put on an ounce. Excited by what I had heard, I wanted to check into a hospital that moment. But it was 11:30 p.m. Too late, I thought, envisioning myself lying on an operating table and undergoing a metamorphosis of Kafkaesque proportions. For people like me, the operation sounded like a promise of a permanent cure for an otherwise incurable disease.

While I was trying to track down an East Coast surgeon skilled in the ways of bypass surgery, a Twiggy-looking friend, who turns thumbs down on everything, launched into a tirade. Her favorite expression is "Hold it! Hold it! Don't you ever look before you leap?" I thought, there she goes again. "Don't you think you ought to do some checking first?" Despite my manner, I knew she was right, so before doing anything rash, I settled down to some serious investigating. I began to think about the nuts and bolts of the surgery. What exactly is a bypass? How long does the operation take? What exactly do they do? How much weight would I lose initially? That was a crucial question. Would there be any complications? Where was it being done in New York?

I called the New York Public Library. After getting a busy signal for an hour and a half and being put on hold for another 25 minutes, a reference librarian—anxious, frenetic, brusque—told me the question was too complicated to answer by phone. "Calls are limited to three minutes," she added, hanging up before I could ask why. When I called the New York Academy of Medicine, a storehouse of medical information, I was told the librarians could not answer medical questions. It was a strange system, I thought, for a medical library. But then, I suppose because the people answering the phones are librarians and not physicians, the people making the rules want to protect the public against misinformation. Maybe they just want to protect themselves from something. Maybe they're just afraid of a malpractice suit. Whatever the reason for it, it's infuriating when you're at a crossroads in your life, trying to make an important decision like a bypass, to have to scrounge for information.

Finally, at the library I consulted a medical dictionary, I learned that in a bypass, the small intestine is severed at one end and attached at another. Well, that didn't sound complicated. Snip here and attach there. What could be easier? What they were talking about was shortening the small intestine. By shortening it, I guess it meant that not only wouldn't you have to eat as much, but you'd never be hungry. It sounded terrific.

When I left the library, I was in high spirits. This is the answer, I thought. This is really going to work. What a break for fat people like me. This is what we've been waiting for all our lives. As I walked past the guard, through a double pair of doors, down a short flight of steps, out onto the street, I suddenly felt a twinge of anxiety. What about the pain? Like most men, when it comes to physical pain, I'm a coward. I said to myself, "Hold it! Hold it! Don't panic.

Don't go to pieces right here on the street, for Christ's sake. Calm down and think things through." My Twiggy friend was right about me, I thought. I'm too damn impulsive. So what if there is a little discomfort? Anyway, if it means I'll be diet-free for the rest of my life, I could live with a little discomfort. Besides, with today's genius surgeons, those dazzling pioneers of organ transplants, artificial hearts, and test-tube babies, if they can create life, certainly it would be painless. I bet there wouldn't even be a scar. Although never having done a beach blanket movie, I didn't care about a little scar—certainly not there.

At a cocktail party, I met a doctor and asked him questions about this operation. He seemed to know something about it.

"Of course, you would have to live with half an intestine or maybe less, depending upon how much they cut. The more they cut away, the better it is for losing weight," he said.

Oh, I thought. That's why they do that. So, instead of having 23 feet of small intestine, I might end up with four or five feet or maybe no intestine.

"Can a person manage on so little?" I asked.

"That's what they're trying to find out."

"What do you mean, that's what they're trying to find out?"

"Well, it's still experimental. They don't know how much to cut yet for the most weight loss." I could feel myself tighten up.

"Incidentally, I don't do that operation. I'm in cardiology."

While I sat around trying to digest all this, I began to brood about my small intestine, thinking what happens to the rest of it? What happens to the part the surgeons don't want? Is it cut out and thrown away, or is it left there in the abdominal cavity to atrophy and die. If I were to have such an operation, I thought, I would always agonize over my small intestine. Being a sentimentalist, I would worry about what it was doing in there, lying limp and lifeless, curling in around itself, waiting for nourishment it would never get. But maybe that was the bargain I would have to make. Maybe I would have to sacrifice a part of myself for that new image.

Later, I found out that the bowel is shortened in such a way that, if it had to be, the whole procedure could be reversed. Reversed? What the hell did that mean? I asked myself. That would mean they would whittle away at me twice? The thought of going under the knife a second time, just to have something corrected? That gave me quite a jolt.

Then I talked to a movie producer I know who had had such an operation. He was miserable. He had diarrhea for a whole year. Puzzled, I wondered why.

"A year is a long time for diarrhea, isn't it?"

"Yeah," he responded.

"Why is that?" I said.

"Why is what?" he said.

"The diarrhea?"

"It's from the operation," he answered.

"I know," I said, "but why?"

"How do I know why?" He was getting irritated. "It's something about a short intestine."

"Oh," I said.

Later I talked to someone else who had had the operation. As we talked, she kept rubbing her abdomen. It was like a nervous tic. Watching her, mesmerized by that involuntary gesture, I thought to myself, "This woman is on the verge of a nervous breakdown."

"Whatever you do," she said, "don't ever have that operation. It's the pits."

"Why," I asked.

"Because you have to spend all your time on the toilet, that's why. Everything goes right through you. You have absolutely no control over your bowels. The diarrhea is intolerable."

As she left, still rubbing, I noticed that she limped slightly on her right side. Was that from the surgery? I thought. The *Los Angeles Times* ran a story about a patient, who as a result of a bypass operation, had become quite ill. Because she was suffering such pain, she tried to commit suicide. After hearing all these terrible things, I was beginning to have serious misgivings, so I decided to see a specialist, which is what I should have done in the first place. What he explained was that controlling obesity by surgical bypass is a risky way of losing weight because of the terrible side effects.

"The side effects are worse than the disease," he said. "For one thing," he said, "there is persistent diarrhea."

"Oh, yes. That I heard about."

"And did you also hear that even by treating it with massive doses of paregoric for practically the whole first year, the diarrhea can still be a problem? Because some patients find it so intolerable, they have to go back and have the whole thing undone."

"Not just because of the diarrhea?"

"Yes, because of the diarrhea. It's a very big problem. The trouble is that by bypassing most of the intestinal tract, and leaving only a short segment of the intestine functioning, there's nothing to digest the food with. That's what makes you lose the weight, but that's what creates a Pandora's box of trouble. You can lose your hair."

"What hair?" I said.

"For those with hair. And you can have nausea and vomiting. You can develop kidney stones and inflammation of the gall bladder which may mean more surgery. You're vulnerable to infections . . . all sorts of things."

"It is a Pandora's box, isn't it?"

"It sure is. Maybe it's okay for the morbidly obese, people who are 500 pounds and over, who would otherwise die from the complications of obesity, but otherwise it's not something you play around with. I know two people who have died from it. They had liver failure. That's the worst complication from all this." Liver failure is irreversible. Once that happens, bypass patients have to have regular liver biopsies to make sure the liver doesn't konk out on them. That's what happened to Betty Hughes, the wife of the ex-governor of New Jersey. After trying for years to lose on various diets, she had a bypass. Well, immediately she developed all the classic symptoms: the diarrhea, the nausea, dehydration, and she lost her hair. When she began to have liver failure, she was rushed to the hospital. After being in a coma for several weeks and fed intravenously the bypass was reversed to save her life. She was lucky. She survived. Others didn't.

"The irony of all this," he said, "is that after going through that nightmare, you can still plateau."

"Plateau? That's a word no dieter likes to hear, Doctor."

"Well, that's the way it is. After the big weight drop the first year, a bypass patient can plateau just like any other dieter. And if he wants to continue losing, he has to go right back to dieting again. It doesn't seem worth it, does it?"

I agreed. As I sat there I thought, I can't believe it. After giving up a part of myself, losing the use of four-fifths of my intestine, suffering damaging diarrhea, risking all the other complications, not to mention my life, I could still plateau. I would still have to diet.

There was no way I would ever consider anything like that, nor would I recommend it to anybody. On the way home, mulling over what my doctor had said about it all, I thought, "Well, it was a terrific idea, it just didn't work." Dieting is tough.

3. Discovering Durham

After years of flop diets, moving between svelte and fat, constantly rummaging through my wardrobe for something to wear, I was desperate again. At times, carried away by the dream of success, I gave away all my "fat" clothes, only to regain the weight and later beg them back. At one time, my wardrobe consisted of clothes in seven different sizes, from 38 to 50. Living in a typical city apartment with barely enough closet space, I would either have to permanently lose weight or open a second-hand clothing store. I had gone through the protein–no starch diet, the starch–no protein diet, the high-fat, the low-fat, the water diet. I was at the end of my rope.

As I waited for the next miracle to come down the pike, I got a call offering me the part of Sancho Panza in the movie *Man of La Mancha*. It was based on the story of the chivalrous visionary Don Quixote de la Mancha, a novel by the seventeenth-century Spanish novelist Miguel de Cervantes, which was to be filmed on location in Rome. I threw some clothes in a suitcase and left town.

Starring in the film was Peter O'Toole, that gaunt, wild, convivial actor, amateur archeologist, bon vivant, jack of all trades and master of all, accomplished horseman, and one of those enviable men who can eat anything anytime and never put on an ounce. Also starring was the legendary Sophia Loren, also known as voluptuous, aloof, tempestuous, vulnerable, shy, maternal, bawdy, sex symbol, earth goddess, equipped with legs that never seem to end, devoted mother, card player, and pasta lover. She lived up to her reputation.

It was my first trip to Italy. As an Italian-American I must at some time or other have considered going to Italy for the very obvious ethnic reasons, but to be suddenly transported there in a Hollywood-style movie with two superstars like O'Toole and Loren was an undreamed-of bonanza. I couldn't have planned it better.

Like the typical tourist, I moved into the world of Roman ruins, gasped at the sight of the Colosseum, stared at the sad-looking Colosseum cats, gawked at the splendors of St. Peter's, and marveled at the serenity of Michelangelo's youthful Pietà. For nine glorious months I forgot about diets and dieting and wallowed in an orgy of eating like a Felliniesque *Dolce Vita* hedonist, gorging on Roman specialties hitherto unfamiliar to the provincial world of a Sicilian from the Bronx.

Whether eating in a small trattoria, a flashy tourist trap, a fashionable chic restaurant, on the movie set, or eating in Sophia's sumptuous palazzo overlooking the Colosseum, Rome was a culinary adventure. In Rome, eating and cooking is a passion and an art, even when it's a simple tomato-mozzarella salad dressed with olive oil and flavored with basil. Unlike the plastic-wrapped supermarket tomatoes in the States, Italian tomatoes are generally vine-ripened by the warm Italian sun with the deep red color and smooth skin texture that have nearly disappeared from American vegetable stalls. Another dish was *Carciofi alla giudea,* young Roman artichokes, trimmed, flattened, and fried to a golden brown. We had spaghetti and white truffles in *Il Topo,* a famous restaurant in the Trastevere section across the Tiber. When the waiter, grating the white truffle onto the spaghetti, said, *"Dica quando* (say when)," I never said it. We ate a sweet spaghetti with baby clam sauce just fished from the sea in an open-air restaurant along the pier in the ancient port of Ostia. The array of fresh antipasti; the mortadella, the gargantuan larded Bolognese pork sausage with its superfine smooth texture; the bite-size *bocconcini,* individual portions of fresh mozzarella cheese; chocolate tartuffe, a triple-chocolate ice cream at *Tre Scalini,* a tourist restaurant in the Piazza Navona facing a Bernini fountain; and the most celebrated of Roman specialties, Roman *abbacchio,* milk-fed baby lamb flavored with sage, rosemary, garlic, and anchovies. Rome was a garden of delights. Romans have a flair for cooking. During their leisurely two-hour lunches—a tradition in Italy—businesses stop for the ritual of eating.

A passionate cook and the author of a recent cookbook, *To Sophia with Love,* Sophia frequently brought homemade food to the set or occasionally prepared a pasta lunch herself, throwing together a simple sauce made with fresh tomatoes and seasoned with basil in less than ten minutes.

Even Peter O'Toole's chauffeur could cook up a delicious pasta and for an afternoon snack once made an unusual tuna sauce.

While I was wallowing in this excess of eating, my girth increased, barely concealed behind the burlap gunnysack costumes. Though it was ideal for my character, the excess weight was pure hell for my sweet donkey Teresa, a placid, docile, fragile creature, too fragile—I thought—to carry around a heavy American actor. I'm terrified of animals anyway. It was agony for me the first time, getting on Teresa. According to Arthur Hiller, the director, my early scenes on Teresa had to be redone because I had such a terrified expression on my face. Though the cast and crew reassured me that donkeys were born beasts of burden, accustomed to carrying even whole houses on their backs, I was not convinced. I was scared stiff. I was afraid she might collapse. Whenever I climbed the tiny portable steps to mount the saddle I would hear a low grunt from Teresa. And as I grew in size her grunts grew louder, until one long day of shooting on the set as I sat waiting around, Teresa slowly began sinking to her knees, completely collapsing under the strain. Fortunately, she had two understudies. The cast and crew were amused. I was humiliated. I was so chagrined that I ran out and bought a box of *amaretti* and hand-fed her to make amends. And she ate and rested while they rushed on her two understudies.

Before the Roman orgy had spent itself, I had gained 50 pounds, tipping the scales at 305. Back home again, at my highest weight ever, I knew I had to do something. I couldn't walk around New York in Sancho Panza gunny sacks. At a total loss again, I heard somehow that that funny man, Buddy Hackett, had been on a rice diet and had had spectacular results with it.

So I immediately put through an SOS to Hackett in California to get the lowdown on the rice diet.

"Listen, Buddy," I said, "I understand—"

Before I could finish my sentence Buddy interrupted.

"Yeah," he said. "I been on the rice diet. You won't like it."

"Why not?"

"Too much rice. Washed out. Rinsed out. Scoured salt-free, three times a day in the beginning. Rice. They put it through the wringer before you get it. And you got to have a urine analysis every morning."

"Why?"

"To check your urine."

"Why?"

"To find out if you been cheating."

"What are you talking about?"

"If you been cheating there'll be salt in your urine and they yell at ya."

"Oh, come on, Buddy."

"I mean it. That's what all those brown paper bags are for."

"What brown paper bags?"

"The brown paper bags the ricers carry around in the morning. It's urine samples. They have to drop them off at the hospital every morning for urine analysis."

Oh, God, I thought. I can't live like that.

"Somebody could make a fortune black-marketing diuretics down there."

"Down where?"

"In Durham, North Carolina. That's where the diet is. They're scared to death of the rice doctor, Kempner. That's why they take all those diuretics—to flush out the kidneys—and laxatives, too. God forbid there should be a grain of salt in your urine."

"You're kidding. . . . Wait a minute, something's coming back to me. I think I heard somebody say something once about the rice diet, but I thought it was because—I thought it was for people who were really very sick or had kidney ailments or were blind or something."

"Look, if you really want a terrific diet, go to the DRC down there. It's got real food. Three squares a day. It's a 700-calorie diet with real food. It's a helluva lot of eating after three bowls of salt-free rice."

"Yeah?"

"Yeah."

"OK," I said, "so what do I do?"

"Call them. They'll take you. They like fat people down there."

"Where is Durham, North Carolina?" I asked.

"Down south," Hackett said.

"Yeah, I know it's down south, but where?"

"I don't know. Just take a plane. It'll get ya there. They got a terrific golf course near there too."

"I don't play golf."

"Well, there's other things to do. They grow tobacco down there, too. That's what they been doing for more than three hundred years."

"What?"

"Growing tobacco."

"Oh. Well, Buddy, thanks for the tip."

"Yeah. Call me in a couple of months. Let me know how you made out."

"Thanks, Buddy, I'll think about it. What've I got to lose?"

"About a hundred pounds."

Actually, I later heard some pretty hilarious stories about Hackett and the Rice House. After he defected he was reported to have poured salt into the urine bottles and had a truckload of pizzas delivered to the Rice House at lunchtime. With Buddy's prankish sense of humor, I don't know . . . it's always possible. I kinda wish I had been around when it happened.

Anyway, on January 14, 1974, I entered the Dietary Rehabilitation Program at the Duke University Medical Center in Durham, North Carolina. Without realizing it, I was making my own personal diet history that day.

In 1974, the Raleigh-Durham Airport looked like an empty lot. There was one hangar, two airline signs, and no facilities for unloading baggage from the plane. Baggage was unloaded manually as passengers disembarked and was de-

posited on the sidewalk in front of the terminal. Buddy
Hackett was pulling my leg, I thought. I don't see any rolling
tobacco fields. I see a deserted airport with very little
action. Except for the southern climate, it looked as if I had
landed in an uncharted wilderness of the Yukon.

Today, seven airlines fly in and out of Durham. Baggage
is unloaded by hydraulic lifts and transferred onto a conveyor belt. An Eastern Airlines Ionosphere lounge decorated in the Art-Deco style of the 1930s (in mauve-pinks and
blues) looks like a Jean Harlow movie set. But that first
time, I wasn't impressed with Durham. This can't be a diet
town, I muttered to myself. There's nobody around. As I
got to know Durham I changed my mind.

The Dietary Rehabilitation Clinic, a division of the Department of Community Health Sciences of the Duke University
Medical Center, was located in the Duke University Graduate Center, a nurses' dormitory and office building.

It was at the Diet Clinic that I first met Dr. Gerard J.
Musante, a clinical psychologist and the director of the
behavioral program, who became a major influence in my
struggle with obesity. Casually at first, Dr. Musante and I
developed a professional relationship over the years as we
examined the behavioral and psychological aspects of my
eating problems, inevitably touching on other unresolved
conflicts. In time, Dr. Musante became my diet doctor guru,
therapist, and friend.

For the first two days, the program included registration,
orientation, a medical examination, behavioral evaluation,
and interviews with the medical director, the behavioral
director, and the dietician. They even took humiliating "before"
pictures. (I wasn't around long enough the first time for the
"after" ones.)

New patients had to have a complete medical workup
including x rays, an EKG and, not only routine laboratory
and diagnostic tests, but also a five-hour Glucose Tolerance
Test (GTT) for hyperglycemia—high blood sugar. After
swallowing a thick syrupy sugar drink, I sat on a bench
outside the laboratory for five hours where a beehive of
nurses took diagnostic blood samples every half hour. The
lab looked like a blood bank.

When I was through with the medical evaluation, I had a

final Howard Johnson's fling the night before starting the diet, stuffing myself on fried clams, hot dogs, French fries, and a triple-flavored banana split occasionally pictured on those Howard Johnson's orange-and-blue laminated menus.

Reporting to the Graduate Center at 7:30 the following morning, I started out on a rocky adventure that ended happily, if belatedly. I also met my first diet buddy, Ruth Drucker from Florida. Together we struggled through the rough spots, encouraging each other along the way. For me, the buddy system has always been an important adjunct of any diet regime.

The Dietary Rehabilitation Program emphasized diet, behavior modification, education, and medical supervision.

We followed a simple mandatory regime.

- To weigh in before breakfast
- To keep a weight chart
- To get blood pressure and pulse readings at designated intervals
- To keep a diary of both
- To consult with medical, psychological, behavioral, and dietary staff members, as needed

The diet—a 700-calorie, moderate protein, moderate carbohydrate, low-fat, low-cholesterol, low-sodium regimen—was originally developed in the late 1960s by Professor Siegfried Heyden, M.D., professor at Duke University.

> Breakfast 150
> Lunch 150
> Dinner 400

I bought a pocket calculator and started counting.

Weighed, measured, and prepared by the Graduate Center Dining Hall Staff, the meals were served cafeteria style, which I never liked. Salt shakers were banished from the dining room. Potassium salt substitutes were used in place of table salt. Posted on the dining room walls were placards with behavior-modification slogans:

- Eat slowly
- Wait twenty seconds before each bite
- Put down your fork after every bite

Since I could never put down any utensil for more than twenty seconds, the placards didn't work for me.

The egg white did.

A menu staple, egg-white omelets were a novelty and a revelation. As is well known, the yolk contains saturated fat and cholesterol, while the egg white is pure protein. According to a catchy Durham slogan, "Egg white is as pure as mother's milk" and only 15 calories per egg.

For breakfast, I preferred an egg-white omelet, plain or with ¼ cup of cottage cheese or half a banana. Rarely did I have a high-carbohydrate, dry cereal breakfast. My personal experience was that I lost more quickly eating an egg-white breakfast. I cooked them at home, using a Teflon nonstick pan to which I add a teaspoon of margarine for taste. A teaspoon of margarine keeps the calorie count down while enhancing the flavor. For me, egg whites did the trick.

A simple exercise program was combined with the menu plan—walking at least two miles a day. Though it's not what they had in mind, I did most of my walking browsing through the shopping malls. The behavioral program included group therapy sessions to examine food-related problems and private therapy for those who wanted it. Most of the time, I just skipped group. Sitting around discussing my eating problems seemed like a pointless intellectual exercise. I knew what my problem was. I overate, I was a chronic binger, and I couldn't stay away from ethnic foods. Besides, it was more fun at the malls. Besides all that there were lectures and videotapes of one sort or another, patient education—all part of the reconditioning process.

It was very much like being back in school—the lectures, the videotapes—learning about nutrition and exercise, finding out what behavior modification was all about, attending group therapy sessions. It's mind-boggling at first, how much information they try to cram down your throat. In time, it all falls into place.

Lecture series were on various topics: "Fats in the Diet," "Smoking and Health," "Cholesterol." Ironically, I happened to catch a scary lecture called "Fats in the Diet," on the risk factors of saturated fats. The lecture included color slides and charts and blue lines and red lines and black lines, criss-crossing each other. Each line representing a significant statistic. When a slide, projected onto the screen, turned out to be the fat-encrusted heart of a 600-pound ex-patient who had died of an overdose of fat, I left the lecture hall.

I skipped the lecture on smoking altogether. Unable to quit smoking at the time, I thought, "Why bother?" I knew what they were going to say. Besides, I wanted to pick up a new sweatsuit at J. C. Penney's. They were having a sale. Frankly, I was never a model pupil either at DRC or later at Structure House.

Though I kept a meticulous diary as directed, even noting daily activities and mood swings, I paid very little attention to the overall program. Partly for show and partly, I suppose, out of a natural curiosity, I would occasionally drop in on a lecture or watch a few minutes of a behavior modification tape. Unconsciously, I began picking up bits and pieces of information that would become the cornerstone of a whole new lifestyle. In time, I realized that it made perfect sense to know the nutritional values of foods, to learn what's in a banana or why too much salt is bad for you or to discover that a potato shell has only fifteen calories.

But in the beginning, I didn't have time for all the extracurricular activity. I was a fat man in a hurry. I wasn't there to attend classes or listen to lectures. I was there to take off one hundred pounds, to trim down to a svelte 205—fast. I wasn't there to listen to somebody talk all day. I didn't want a master's degree in Health Ed. I wanted magic. Abracadabra. Puff! Now you see it, now you don't.

But Dr. Gerard J. Musante is no magician. He practices no sleight-of-hand. He has no tricks up his sleeve. As a clinical psychologist, trained in behavior therapy and specializing in obesity problems, Musante warned early on against unrealistic expectations and preached that only through long-term behavioral changes could permanent weight loss be achieved. But I was too busy counting calories and charting a downward curve on my weight chart to get the message.

And when I wasn't counting calories, I was running around Durham, sightseeing, browsing through the malls, window-shopping, antiquing, and going to the movies almost every other night. I saw more clinkers in Durham, North Carolina, than any other place in the world.

Once, on my way to the movies, I spotted a heavy "ricer" sitting in the hotel lobby almost catatonic-looking, popping Raisinets into his mouth one at a time with unfailing precision. I couldn't take my eyes off him. Remaining outwardly motionless, except for the steady movement of the jaw and the perpetual motion of the arm, proceeding in relays from elbow to wrist to hand to mouth with expert marksmanship. Fascinated, I started to keep score, but when the number climbed to 110, I ran out of time and had to leave. Whatever the odds were that he would break the candy habit, the likelihood of his ever giving up chocolate-covered raisins seemed doubtful. He was still popping when I left for the movies. I picked up a packet of Trident sugarless gum along the way but I kept dreaming of popping Raisinets.

But I saw other things, too. I saw the Gothic architecture of Duke University endowed in 1924 by James Buchanan Duke, the tobacco heir; the Chapel Tower is patterned after the famous Bell Harry Tower of Canterbury Cathedral. I saw the Duke Gardens, with its terraced landscaping and wisteria-covered pergola. The centerpiece is a pretty lily pond. I saw the jutting concrete-and-glass Burroughs-Wellcome Research Building designed by architect Paul Rudolph. And I saw the old pink brick tobacco warehouses with their funny little crenelated chimneys near downtown Durham, many of which today are being converted into condominiums and open markets. I saw the blossoming magnolias with their fragrant white flowers and visited the factory of the American Tobacco Company where I got a free sample of nonmentholated cigarettes. And I listened to the sound of the freight train of the Southern Railway that went on for miles and miles as it cut across Durham, connecting North and South. The rhythmic clacking sound of the wheels and the whistle sounding steadily as it went by were romantic reminders of the past.

I even watched the dance-hungry dieters at the wild Tuesday-night disco at the Ramada Inn Downtown. Uninhibited, in an atmosphere of acceptance, they pack onto the crowded dance floor, throwing themselves into a frenzy of dancing. Under the strobe lights, they contort their bodies into the jerky movement of rock, stomping their heavy feet to the shrill, earsplitting disco beat, having a wonderful time. In many posh metropolitan discos where people sometimes show up in their Bergdorf Goodman finery, fat people often huddle in darkened corners, ashamed and frightened and too embarrassed about the way they look to get out on the dance floor. In Durham, they can really say, "Move over." Unlike anyplace else that I know of, fat people can appear publicly in a sweat suit, shorts, or an outsized bikini and jump into the motel pool feeling free and accepted.

There was one day I will never forget—when a certain patient walked into group absolutely euphoric. I thought she was stoned. I thought she must have had a chocolate bar and gone into sugar shock. Suddenly, she snapped out of it, whirling herself around, like a would-be Isadora Duncan, letting out a shriek that echoed through the corridors and reached clear out to the far end of the parking lot. Then just as quickly, her mood shifted again. This time she became almost catatonic. For a count of ten, she remained motionless and rigid—in a state of suspended animation—until slowly, almost imperceptibly, she drew herself up, and assuming an almost regal stance, prepared to speak. With a look of ecstasy on her face, she faced the group and in a hushed whisper said, "I'm cured. I have found the answer. I'll never have to worry about dieting again."

There was dead silence. Nobody moved. Everybody froze. We were spellbound, waiting for the denouement. To a group of die-hard dieters always on the lookout for the answer, that was an earth-shattering statement.

I heard someone in the back say, "What did she say?"

"She said she's cured," the person next to her answered.

What? How? How could she be cured? somebody else wanted to know.

Suddenly, like a Greek chorus, everybody started whispering to each other—chanting in unison—"She never has to diet again. She's cured. She found the answer."

An aggressive-sounding patient in the front shouted, "She must be crazy. How could anybody lick the diet?"

Somebody who obviously agreed with her said, "She just thinks she found the answer."

Then a more even-tempered newcomer piped up, "How do you know? Maybe she has. After all, miracles can happen."

"No, they can't," somebody yelled back at her.

"I don't believe in miracles."

"Neither do I."

"Oh, shut up, Mae. Don't encourage them."

"Well, I don't."

"Mae?!"

She held up her hands. The room quieted down. We all waited with bated breath. She then launched into the story of her great personal revelation. We were on the edge of our seats.

"There are 200 calories in a slice of pizza," she said. "Three pieces of pizza at 200 calories a slice is 600 calories all together. Now, listen to this"—ticking off the numbers on the fingers of her left hand as she spoke—"if I have one slice for breakfast, and one for lunch, and one for dinner, not only would I be within my daily calorie count, but I would also have 100 calories to spare and before going to bed, I can have another half a piece of pizza which adds up to 700 calories." Elated, she looked around at the group waiting for their approval. I think she was about to take a bow.

With that, the spell was broken. It was a long time before anybody in the group could speak. Finally—flabbergasted at what I had just heard—I turned to her and said, "Now, wait a minute. Are you trying to tell me that you're advocating a diet of three slices of pizza a day and half a slice before bedtime?"

"That's right," she said, still on cloud nine.

"What a great idea."

"She's a lunatic."

"Why didn't somebody think of that before?"

"That's about the worst idea I ever heard of. First of all, I'm one of the few fat people who hates pizza."

"I'm going to try it."

"How much protein is there in a pizza?" somebody wanted to know.

"Who cares?"

"She licked the diet?"

"I told you, Mae, next time you won't be so negative."

"Poor girl, she needs another kind of doctor."

Somebody in the back giggled. The giggling turned into hysterical laughter.

"What a minute," I said. "Hold it. Hold it. What are you talking about? Are you crazy? It would never work."

"Why not? Why—why wouldn't it work?" she asked.

"Because nobody can stop at three slices of pizza—ever. That's why. I ought to know."

"He's right," somebody groaned. "Oh, damn. Once a person starts in on a pizza, one slice becomes two, two becomes six. And before you know it, he ends up eating the whole pie."

"And, furthermore," I said, "even if there were any nutritional value in a slice of pizza—which I seriously doubt—how long do you think a person could keep that up before dying of malnutrition? How long do you think a person could live on three slices of pizza a day?"

"At least a day."

"A pizza diet," somebody moaned. "What a terrific idea. What a shame."

As we started to leave, I overheard two women saying under their breath, "Do you suppose the same thing could work with strawberry shortcake? How many calories are there in a strawberry shortcake?"

"With my recipe? A week's supply!"

They were still mulling it over as we left group. Fantasies die hard.

Still, I sympathized with her. I had my own pizza horror story. Once when I was at the Dietary Rehabilitation Clinic, I almost had a mini-breakdown. I had been on the program for about a month when, all of a sudden, I could feel a classic binge coming on, the kind I recognized from way back. I needed a pizza fix.

Whenever I get an uncontrollable urge like that, I really go off the deep end. I become obsessed. Only after I satisfy the craving and get it all out of my system do I finally settle down and come back to my senses. But by that time, it's usually too late. My weight is out of control and on its way to the stratosphere. With my notorious history of uncontrollable binges, I knew that if I once lost control, as I habitually did, that would finish the diet. There's nothing I can do but let it run its course. There I was on a voluntary weight control program that I hoped would save my life and, suddenly, I was about to give up again.

After getting off to a terrific start at the DRC, gaining confidence and gaining strength, I started to weaken again. I had lost forty pounds in four weeks. I thought I had finally found the answer. Buddy Hackett was right, I thought. He knew what he was talking about when he recommended the Dietary Rehabilitation Clinic. The diet worked like a charm. Losing forty pounds in four weeks was a once-in-a-lifetime experience. I loved it and I had visions of dropping another forty before leaving Durham. But because of a weakness for certain ethnic foods and a natural predisposition to uncontrollable binges of psychotic dimensions, I was about to break faith with what I intuitively knew was my last chance. I was panicky. After a lifetime of broken promises to myself, I didn't want to go back on this diet. I wanted it to work. But, when I'm caught in the grip of a psychotic episode—a monomaniacal compulsion like that—there's no hope for me. There's no way I can stop it.

After having gone through all the trouble of finding Durham— practically sending out a search party—scouring the country, checking it out long distance with Buddy Hackett, crying out to the world for help and then traveling 672 miles to a small Southern tobacco town, cutting myself off from family and friends, isolating myself from civilization, practically committing myself to solitary confinement, settling in for an indefinite stay, was I about to blow it all for one lousy pizza?

I was just going to try to ignore the whole thing so I turned on the television set and sat back, waiting for dinnertime, which was only a couple of hours away. What's the first thing that came on the television set? A Pizza Hut commercial. I tripped over myself, running to turn off the set.

So I went straight to Dr. Musante and I leveled with him. I said, "Listen, I have this terrible craving for a pizza. What am I going to do? It's excruciating. Help." Easy and relaxed, Dr. Musante sat back, smiled a minute, and then—totally unruffled by my hysterical outburst and my plaintive cry for help—he started to explain a very basic and underlying principle of the entire diet program. It was the first of such talks—the beginning of a gradual shift in my whole attitude toward diets.

He started in by saying, "Go ahead and have it."

I thought I had gone deaf or something. "Excuse me, Dr. Musante, but I thought I heard you say, 'Go ahead and have it.'"

"That's right. That's what I said. If that's what you want, go ahead and have it." I must have looked at him strangely, because he took one look at me and started to laugh.

"I'm glad you think it's funny," I said. "What do you mean, go ahead and have it? You keep saying that, but I don't know what you're talking about. When was it ever okay to have pizza? That doesn't make any sense."

"You've done very well here. You've lost forty pounds in four weeks. You've been totally structured. You have this craving. You don't think that if you wait fifteen or twenty minutes, this craving will go away?"

"No."

"Okay. You mean, if you find a substitute, like maybe going shopping for a new pair of sneakers or something . . ."

"No."

"Well, then have it. And don't feel guilty about it."

Losing weight, he added, does not mean you will never ever be unstructured again. That's not the way the diet works. You will be unstructured. It's going to happen, but there's nothing unnatural about that. Diets are meant to be broken—if you do it right. Plan your unstructured eating into your overall menu plan and go right back to structured eating when you get it all out of your system. That's the key. If one day you have a chocolate bar, or pie a la mode, or French fries, it does not mean you've blown the diet.

Planned unstructured eating is an ideal way to handle those occasional times when you need to satisfy a craving for something. Self-denial is not the answer. Structure's the answer.

Of course, if it becomes a habit, that is, if planned unstructured eating becomes a way of life and is really masking unstructured eating, that's something else. You'll be able to tell the difference in time, he said.

There are some people who cannot handle prolonged deprivation. They look for gimmicks and loopholes; they can misuse the structured binge.

Dieting is not easy. There is no short cut. It takes

stamina. It takes courage. It takes dogged determination. And it takes the will to win. It also takes a lot of planning and thought.

After that meeting with Dr. Musante, I began to get an inkling that there was more to this dieting business than the numbers game. For a long time, it was the only game in town. Counting calories was important to be sure, but other things were equally important. In the beginning, I was too busy losing pounds to care about anything else. I wasn't interested in concepts. Who had time for concepts? I had too much weight to lose. When you're over a hundred pounds overweight, you want action, not words. But the talk with Musante that day struck a chord. He had put a bug in my ear. Even though it would take a long time to take hold, it was a beginning. When we were through, I felt a whole lot better about the diet and a whole lot better about myself.

Properly understood and correctly used, a planned binge can also help to get rid of a lot of aggression, he said. Whenever someone is on a restricted diet for any length of time, there's bound to be a lot of pent-up anger and frustration, a gnawing feeling of deprivation. There's no way of avoiding those negative feelings. They are part and parcel of the whole dieting process. A structured binge can help neutralize those feelings of rage and anger and smooth the way for the long haul, too.

Although it took me seven years to completely assimilate this basic principle, in the end it paid off in a big way. It started at DRC and ended up all the way home. Today, when I get a craving for something—a hero sandwich, Southern fried chicken, spareribs, or any other "unstructured" food—I don't panic. I don't fall apart. I have no guilt. Once I get it out of my system, I know I'll go right back to structured eating. Dr. Musante was right. A planned binge is a good thing.

So, that night, with Dr. Musante's words still buzzing in my ears, I made a beeline for the neighborhood pizza parlor. It was somewhere on Main Street in the heart of downtown Durham.

An Italian pizza parlor is always crowded and noisy, like a Fellini carnival. There is always an old-fashioned jukebox in the background, blaring a Sinatra record and the Italian waiters scurrying around like crazy, frantically taking orders in a garbled script, doing their disorganized best to meet the challenge of a full house. Admittedly, it must be rough trying to wait on a roomful of pizza freaks, all clamoring for their food at the same time, screaming for personalized service they never get, demanding individual attention that was nonexistent.

But Italian waiters are unique. They thrive on adversity. They also have a knack for creating havoc and disorder. It's a national characteristic. They are unparalleled paragons of chaos. Nobody can beat them—unless it is the Jewish waiters at the old Stage Delicatessen in New York City. Ordering pastrami on rye at the old Stage Deli is like watching an obstacle race. After a fifty-minute wait, if you are lucky, a blasé, bedraggled, harried, high-handed waiter might show up as he barrels through to the kitchen with his pocket full of back-up orders; or if he seems to cock his ear in your direction or is good at lip reading, he might intuit what you want—assuming, of course, that he can catch a glimpse of your face through the semaphore wig-wagging of hands and arms, all trying to get his disinterested attention.

Eventually, if your luck held out, he might turn up with that hot pastrami and—depending on the mood of the day—it might even land where it was supposed to: in front of you, and not in some stranger's lap at the other end of the table. Nobody I knew was ever that lucky. Of course, if it looked like he was lost for good and you were never going to get out of there, you could always nibble on the sour tomatoes. Today, of course, I know that sour tomatoes are an "unstructured" food because of the salt content. Brine is pure salt and water, but in those days, ignorance was bliss.

Eventually, he would return with that thick, fatty, delicious never-lean pastrami on rye. From then on, I was lost to the world, devouring it down to the last peppercorn. That is my idea of Jewish heaven.

But when it comes to taking pizza orders, there's nobody like an Italian. Like the deli waiters, they take them on the run without stopping for air. Once they have the order in hand, they shout them out across the room, with deafening precision, bouncing them off the walls, pitching them back toward the kitchen within earshot of the poor beleaguered cook, who himself is performing feats of dexterity—flinging his pizza dough high into the air in gyrating motions, catching it deftly in his hands with each downward revolution, sending it right back up again in a continuous succession of whirls. It's not everybody who can juggle a doughy mass with such swinging adroitness. That takes agility and style.

Whenever we'd get a craving for a pizza we'd hop the El and ride three stops to Castle Hill Avenue, a major Italian thoroughfare. That's where all the posh Italian restaurants were, so we thought. Clustered together, among the sidewalk pushcarts and the Italian vendors hawking their wares, was a whole slew of first-rate Italian pizzerias, frequented by pizza fanatics like me. We'd pick a spot—order six pizzas at a time—and dig into an orgy of combinations, ranging from the simple to the elaborate: plain, with or without green pepper, mushroom, sausage. In those carefree days, we had a lot of fun growing up. Sometimes after polishing off the six pizzas, we'd sit around for hours, just gabbing about nothing in particular, feasting our eyes on Rita Hayworth lookalikes (wondering if we would "get lucky"), soaking in the atmosphere, storing up the ethnic sights and sounds that we'd cherish later on or forever arguing the merits of Sicilian pizza and Neapolitan pizza. There were partisans on both sides. As everybody probably knows by now, Sicilian pizza is square shaped and 1½″ thick, while the Neapolitan pizza—traditionally better known—has a flat thin crust. It's topped with tomato sauce and mozzarella cheese and garnished with garlic. In the perennial contest between the two, I was always nonpartisan. I could go either way. Sicilian pizza is too rustic for some tastes, not as versatile as the other. For me, it was always a draw.

Of course, while we were developing our tastebuds in that convivial setting and eyeing the specialties of the house, we were also sowing the seed of childhood memories, laying the bedrock of future dreams.

The little things we took for granted then would linger forever, like the old faded murals that decorated the pizzeria walls—the scenes of the Bay of Naples with Mount Vesuvius in the background, erupting or momentarily quiescent, or the primitive-looking painting of the Isle of Capri, or the garish scene of the glorious coastline of Sorrento, bathed in the glaring Mediterranean light. There were also all those schmaltzy Italian songs we used to sing all the time, unmindful of the plaintive cry for a paradise lost in the sentimental words of "O, Sole Mio," and "Take Me Back to Sorrento." We were second-generation American, what did we know? And then there was the fleeting glimpse of the itinerant musician, lugging his heavy accordion around, constantly having to hitch it back up on his shoulder, where it would slide off from the weight, as he made his way to his next engagement, conveniently at the pizzeria around the corner. Finally—there is the distant echo of the mandolin.

Now, I have no intention of evoking the stereotype of the Italian organ grinder or of Guido, the Italian waiter with the handlebar mustache and his large white apron. That's something else again. I'm talking about roots. To me a pizzeria is a very nostalgic place. It's home. It's where I grew up. It's where I belong.

Unlike its Italian counterpart in the Bronx, a Southern pizza parlor is very, very different. It's a cross between a storefront restaurant and a fast food snack bar. The one in Durham was small, overlit, with neon lights, a handful of empty tables, and a fast-food menu that included chilidogs, donuts, Southern fried chicken, and even hominy grits. There were no Italian waiters, just one waitress.

However different a Southern pizzeria may seem to us Northerners, it's still a pizzeria. So when the pretty, blond Southern waitress sauntered over in her wistful, lilting, casual Southern way, all in her own good time, smiling from ear to ear, I immediately said, "I'd like a pizza, please."

She slowly took out her pad, having misplaced her pencil, she sauntered back to the counter, looked under the counter, looked in the cash register, and finally found this stub of a pencil, behind the napkin holder.

She sauntered over to me again. "What kind would you like?" The pause seemed interminable.

"What kind have you got?" I said.

"All kinds: olives, onions, mushrooms, that Italian sausage, salami, cheese . . ." I fully expected her to tell me she had some with black-eyed peas and hominy grits.

"I'll tell you what. I'll just have it plain with mozzarella."

She stopped in the middle of her writing. "Mozzarella, is that that stringy stuff?"

"That's right," I said.

She smiled sweetly. "Mozzarella? Is that what it's called?" She tried to write it down. "Well, we just call it stringy cheese."

"How long will that take?" I asked, looking around at the empty tables.

"Well, that depends," she said.

"On what?"

"On how long it takes for the oven to heat. It's been so hot today. We've been very slow. Nobody seems to want pizza today, except you. So we'll just have to start it up."

She suggested I take a long walk around the block until it was ready.

So I took her advice and did some window shopping nearby. It was too late to buy anything. All the stores were closed by then. So I window shopped, watching the clock— killing time—which is exactly what I didn't want to do. It was very hot. She was right. It was a particularly hot day in Durham. It was not a day for browsing, especially if you were famished. I was wilting. It was cooler in the pizza shop. So I decided to go back.

When I got there, I saw a skinny kid at the counter eating a chilidog. I wondered if I should switch. Under the circumstances, it seemed like the smart thing to do.

But I stuck it out, waiting for the big moment when she'd bring me my pizza. It took a long time. I thought it would never happen. Finally, I saw her walking toward me with a big white pizza box in her hand. She placed it on the counter and started to tie it up with white string. I knew this was going to take at least another forty-five minutes. "Don't bother. I'll do it myself." Once I'd tied the box and paid my bill, I headed back to the hotel.

While I was waiting for the elevator to take me up to my room, I suddenly heard a whole group of dieters come traipsing in. I wanted to eat my pizza. I didn't want to be disturbed and now I had to face the whole of the DRC holding a pizza box in my hand. There is no disguising a pizza box. A pizza box is definitely a pizza box. It doesn't contain a hat. It doesn't contain jewelry. It doesn't contain clothing. It contains the forbidden pizza.

They said nothing. Nobody commented. They just stared at me. But I knew what they were thinking:

"Imagine."

"No control."

"Unbelievable."

"He's as fat as a house."

"He'll never make it."

"Why does he bother?"

"Why doesn't he just leave?"

The trip seemed interminable. We finally got to the seventh floor. I thought we'd never get there.

Then, by some quirk of modern technology, the elevator malfunctioned. It skipped or jumped or did something—I don't know—some crazy unexpected jerking motion. I had been holding the pizza box from underneath and as the elevator lurched, I reached for the box in an effort to protect it. In the same jerking moment, I grabbed it by the string. It broke and the whole thing splattered to the floor, splashing tomato sauce and stringy cheese all over everybody. It was humiliating. I did my best to make amends: I apologized all over the place, trying to wipe people clean with whatever I could find in my pocket. As the door opened at my floor, I scooped up the whole mess—still apologizing as I got out—and dumped it all in a nearby trash can. The last thing I heard when the door closed behind me was:

"Poor thing. He tried to cheat and look what happened."

Once I got to my room, I breathed a sigh of relief. Peace and quiet at last. Then a miraculous thing happened. I lost the urge for pizza. Maybe it was the memory of pizza splattered on the elevator floor, covered with dust and dirt—whatever it was, I lost the desire for it. Maybe Dr. Musante was right. If you wait fifteen or twenty minutes, you'll lose the urge.

Suddenly I got hysterical thinking about the whole incident. I could not stop laughing for the rest of the night. I laughed myself to sleep.

Actually, it had all turned out for the best. When I stepped on the scale the next morning, I had dropped another pound. Losing a whole pound more than compensated for the loss of that ill-fated pizza. I remember calling my friends and telling the story. It went so well I told it on the Carson show.

I must interject something here. I am very fortunate in having extraordinarily loyal and loving friends. Recently, I lost one, Dolly Jonah, a friend for over twenty-five years, who was married to Will Holt, a gifted writer, lyricist, and composer.

It was traditional to spend Thanksgiving with the Holts—a tradition that started because many of our friends come from other parts of the country. Dolly and Will decided that no one would ever spend Thanksgiving "away from home." She was one of the great cooks, and she would spend days preparing the foods we loved: a cranberry mold, turkey stuffed with fruits, nuts, and blended with meats and carefully chosen herbs and spices. Will, who had his own specialties, would prepare the delectable vegetables. I, of course, was in charge of desserts.

Though I am a native New Yorker and have family here, it was understood that I was also part of the Holt family. My sister, who I am sure would have preferred I spend Thanksgiving with her, never interfered. She adored Dolly and Will and understood. Even after they had a son, Courtney—now sixteen years old—the Holts continued the tradition. Courtney grew up celebrating Thanksgiving with a very large "family."

Dolly was sympathetic about my weight problem. (She always had five pounds to lose. "It's all relative," she would say. "My losing five pounds is as important as your forty or fifty.") Once, on a shopping spree, when we were both dieting—and on that particular day, starving—we made a pact not to mention food for the rest of the day. We were succeeding beautifully. I commented on our dentist and how pretty his wife was. Dolly said, "Really? I've never met his linguine." "You never met his *what*?!" I howled. "Oh, my God," she screamed. "All I've been thinking about for the last two hours is linguine with clam sauce." Doubled up with laughter, we both collapsed in front of Bloomingdale's on 59th Street and Lexington Avenue. A passerby commented to her friend, "Look at them. Drunk at this hour. It's a disgrace." That only made matters worse, of course. We struggled to help each other up for what seemed like hours.

Dolly was an actress. A rare and wonderful actress. She was also a rare and wonderful person. There will be Dolly Jonah stories told within our circle of friends forever. I miss her greatly. I know she knows that.

Anyway, for years Durham was a haven and a retreat for me, a place to cool off from the battering city pressures and to unwind from the coilspring of theatrical tensions.

Actors lead troubled lives. Chronically unemployed, tormented by self-doubt, beset with insecurity, actors live in a frenzy of hysteria and despair. They are either feted or ignored, despised or adored, battered or pampered. They inhabit a world that turns on whim and fancy and a lot of luck, living on the ragged edge of disaster in stultifying deprivation.

Trying to survive, some actors threaten to commit suicide with manic regularity; others get by with vodka martinis dreaming of standing ovations. Even with a streak of madness, there is very little chance of survival for most.

For most actors, it's a waiting game. Some wait with good humor, others with rancor. Some tilt at windmills, but most stab hopelessly at success in last-ditch efforts to score. They wait in the unemployment line, they wait for an agent to call; they wait for that once-in-a-lifetime part, for Lady Luck, for the telephone to ring, mocking that ugly overworked "Don't call me, I'll call you." They wait for the *Playboy* interview, a television series, the kleig lights, the cover story, the big contract, the talk shows, the limo, the autograph collectors, the name above the title. They wait for dreams, for hope, for success, for acceptance, for love. Sometimes I think we're all waiting for Godot.

In Durham, I can sometimes get away from it all—not for long, but for a few weeks at a time, giving my jangled nerves a chance to repair. I think that's why I enjoyed going as frequently as I did. I could escape.

Providing, that is, I wouldn't have to interrupt my treatment for a job offer or a family crisis or a medical emergency or anything else surprising that might come up. Taking off for a job at a moment's notice—if one is lucky enough to be working—is symptomatic of an actor's lifestyle. An actor might be off on a summer package or on a road company of a Broadway play, an out-of-town tryout, a television show in California, a movie in Rome. Traveling is part of the job.

Even during that wonderful first trip to Durham, when I lost forty pounds in four weeks, I was suddenly called away for a medical emergency. Another time I had to leave for a Carol Burnett show.

And once I had just arrived to continue my treatment when my agent called, saying, "You have a movie offer. Could you leave immediately?"

"Wait a minute," I screamed. "I just got here."

"You had better leave immediately," he repeated.

"What do you mean I better leave immediately?" I shouted back.

"They're waiting for you on the movie set in California."

I left immediately, uncertain again about when I might return.

During another Durham stay, I had to leave for a film in Paris. I didn't mind that too much. Like the proverbial American in Paris, I saw the city from the top of the Eiffel Tower and sampled French cuisine at the legendary Maxim's. The menu looked like a Toulouse-Lautrec poster. The prices were like today's interest rates, but the food was scrumptious. With friends, I shared a sumptuous dinner at Maxim's as we sampled each other's dishes: coquilles Saint-Jacques, poached salmon, a rack of lamb, and raspberries. For me, Maxim's is to Paris what Operakelleron is to Copenhagen, what the Savoy is to London, and what the Excelsior is to Rome. In Venice across the Rialto Bridge there is a small restaurant that makes a delectable shrimp dish called shrimp Madame Bovary. It is not on the menu; you have to know about it and order it specially. It's prepared in a cream sauce with sherry and herbs and cooked *a tavola* in a chafing dish. That was a gustatory high point of a Venetian side trip I took while filming in Paris. An unforgettable taste treat.

In less opulent surroundings, I tasted other traditional French dishes: a cassoulet, a bouillabaisse, a pâté, marrons glacés along the Champs-Élysées. In Paris nobody thinks about weight. At least I didn't. I just ate.

Because of my erratic lifestyle, which with luck will continue indefinitely, I had to make time to squeeze in a Durham visit between jobs. Admittedly, that's not the way to undertake the treatment. For the program to be immediately effective, it's essential to stay for a minimum of four weeks, depending upon a person's goal weight. Unable to do that consistently, my treatment for long periods of time was as erratic as my work schedule. For years it was spotty and incomplete. But despite the gaps, with my own persistence and Dr. Musante's encouragement, I ultimately put it all together. But that didn't happen for years.

As I was getting ready for another trip to Durham, I received some exciting news: I was asked to appear in a production of *The Blue Bird*. I was offered the part of Dog, a plum role in the film. It was the first Soviet-American production ever. The star-studded cast included Elizabeth Taylor, Jane Fonda, Cicely Tyson, and Ava Gardner, and it was to be directed by the legendary George Cukor. I couldn't wait to begin. I never dreamed I would ever see Russia, let alone with Taylor, Fonda, Tyson, and Gardner. How lucky can you get?

4. The (Literal) Growth of an Actor

The trip to the Union of Soviet Socialist Republics was a memorable experience. I still have the battle scars to prove it. At the time—for geopolitical reasons, I suppose—there was no direct flight from New York to the U.S.S.R., and that meant going by a long drawn-out route, a little like taking that slow boat to China.

Despite their loud noises to the contrary, the Soviets have a nose for business, too, and impressed with the prospect of a joint Soviet-American film venture and with a little prodding by Edward Lewis, the film's executive producer, the Russians agreed to have my visa ready in time for my departure. When it comes to paper work, the Russians have been known to linger and languish and keep their supplicants on hold for eternity. Deadlines is not a word they understand. I think it's because our alphabets are different.

With only about a week to go before the scheduled flight, the Russians advised us to pick up our visas at the Russian Embassy in Washington, D.C. I was excited about doing *The Blue Bird,* and looked forward to visiting Russia and sampling the authentic Russian cuisine, familiar to me (or so I thought) from years of eating in the Russian Tea Room.

The Russian Tea Room is a landmark New York restaurant. From its opening in 1926, it has been frequented by a theatrical crowd—actors, musicians, dancers, writers, artists, and agents.

Theatrical deals are made and consummated at the Russian Tea Room. I signed my contract for the "Lily Tomlin

Special" there, over a triple order of strawberries Romanoff which splattered on page three as I was licking off the spoon. Fortunately, it did not obscure my signature, and in no way invalidated the contract.

I have developed a taste for Russian food, nurtured right there on 57th Street at the Russian Tea Room. I was looking forward to sampling all those traditional Russian dishes. I love their boiled beef with horseradish sauce, their red cabbage and their Eggplant Orientale, a zesty eggplant appetizer, and their blini with caviar. Every Wednesday, they prepare the famous Russian Pelmeni, a Siberian dumpling filled with chopped meat and served in a meat broth garnished with sour cream. It has a famous Cossack history.

And then, of course, there's caviar.

When I was growing up, I always thought caviar was one of the seven wonders of the world. Now that I'm older, I know it is. Like many of my friends, I am addicted to Russian caviar, especially the crème de la crème of Russian caviars: the fresh whole grain Beluga malossol caviar—the kind that is absolutely cost-prohibitive. Although pressed caviar is just as good, I still prefer the whole grain, pearly gray "berries," from the giant Beluga.

Once on a gluttonous rampage, I bought a whole pound of fresh Beluga from Zabar's, the famous gourmet delicatessen on Broadway and 80th Street. That day, after leaving Zabar's, alone in my kitchen, leaning at a tilt on the refrigerator door, spooning the caviar right out of the jar, I gobbled it up in one continuous burst of physical energy. With my finger, I gingerly scraped out the last precious grain caught in the fold of the jar.

Anticipating unlimited quantities of this precious food, at rock-bottom prices, I began to think of the Soviet Union as another land of milk and honey. I couldn't wait to get over there. I was going to go hog wild on their caviar. In the meantime, I had about a week to get ready. There was a lot of last-minute shopping to do. Unsure of what to bring, I asked people, "Have you ever been to Russia?" I always got a different answer. One person said, "Now, don't forget, you must bring your own toilet paper." Somebody else said, "Now, remember, you'll need overshoes." Another person said, "Don't bother with hats. You can get great fur hats in

Russia—dirt cheap." So I scratched hats from the shopping list. Somebody even said, "Well, I've never been there myself, but I've heard that you can't get a pen." That stumped me.

We had a rendezvous with the Russian Embassy. With a minimum of fanfare and absolutely no red tape, our visas were ready when we arrived. If there were any truth to the rumor that Brezhnev himself had ordered the Russians to roll out the red carpet, I never knew, but everything was in tip-top shape with the proper authorities, our papers were stamped, and in no time, we were escorted out, past a roomful of weary-looking people who looked as if they had been waiting around for a long time.

Since the flight was not until 9 p.m., my assistant, Jack Betts, an actor-friend who was between jobs (You may know him as Ivan Kipling in *One Life to Live*), and I checked into the Embassy Hotel, where we had accommodations for the day, courtesy of Twentieth Century-Fox. We spent the rest of the time hitting favorite Washington restaurants. We sampled an appetizer at Mary Lou's, had the main course at O'Donnell's, and finished off with dessert and coffee at John's Coffee House. Before the flight, we even had time for a delicious cup of Irish coffee.

We arrived at the London airport to change planes for Leningrad. According to the airport scuttlebutt, Greta Garbo had just come in from Brussels. Jack was speechless. I made a complete "U" turn, tripped over my left foot, and almost went flat on my face trying to catch a glimpse of her. Tim Wood, director George Cukor's assistant, met us at the airport to help with traveling arrangements, forgot why he was there and went after her, saying "I'd give my eyeteeth for an autograph of Garbo." But he must have remembered her lifelong passion for privacy, made famous by that time-worn message of "wanting to be alone," so he stopped in his tracks, wistfully staring after the immortal screen idol as she simply got lost in the crowd. But out of sight is not out of mind, if Garbo is the object of your affection.

Standing there, I suddenly remembered Garbo's *Ninotchka*, that 1939 Hollywood spoof about a group of Marxists who, once having tasted "la vie Parisienne," flounder ideologically, longing to stray far from home. Irving Berlin wrote about it in his probing how to keep 'em down on the farm after they've seen "Paree."

In the movie, Ninotchka is sent to Paris to check up on the machinations of a trio of Soviet emissaries, sent earlier to sell the court jewels of a former countess for tractor money. Initially humorless and cynical about Paris, Comrade Ninotchka falls under the romantic spell of Paris in the spring. She also falls madly in love with Melvyn Douglas, a debonair capitalist, under whose tutelage she is treated to a heavy dose of capitalist materialism, bound to change anybody's outlook on life. She, too, begins to waver politically, gradually deviating from communist ideology.

There was one scene in the movie that had a special meaning to me: the four woebegone friends have a nostalgic reunion dinner at Ninotchka's flat. Except for a hapless comrade who had accidentally smashed his egg in his pocket, each contributes a precious egg to the collective meal. Whipping up a Parisian-style omelet, the friends reminisce about their carefree days in Paris. In Russia, I would think often about that scene.

It seems to me that in my childhood (being a movie buff), I always remember the eating scenes from films. After seeing *Ninotchka,* omelets seem so glamorous. After all, if Greta Garbo makes an omelet, there's got to be something to it. For years I tried desperately to duplicate the kind of omelet that the elusive Miss Garbo made. Even Scarlett O'Hara biting into a turnip and saying, "I will never be hungry again," made me salivate. Nor will I ever forget the scene in *The Magnificent Ambersons,* in which Tim Holt swallows a strawberry shortcake as Agnes Moorhead was telling him some very important news. I don't remember the news. I do remember the strawberry shortcake.

I don't know whether it was Garbo, the omelet scene, or remembering *The Magnificent Ambersons,* but suddenly I was hungry. There was still time for lunch before the Leningrad flight, so we whipped over to Wheeler's, a popular fish restaurant off Piccadilly Circus, in the heart of London's theater district. Like a homing pigeon, whenever I am in London, I always find my way back to Wheeler's. They make a delicious Dover sole almondine with a light lemon sauce. It's a menu favorite and an excellent diet dish.

Unfortunately, like many other English restaurants, they also make a terrific trifle, an elaborate, not-so-low-calorie, rich, thick, pudding-like dessert. It's made with a sponge cake soaked in sherry and brandy, and layers of different colored custard puddings, filled with fruits and nuts and candy, and topped with heavy double cream. With trifle, the sky's the limit. There can be as many as ten different layers. It is set in a large glass bowl, so the different colors can be seen running together along the sides of the bowl, like a colorful display of summer fireworks.

Jack, who never has to worry about his weight, and who is normally addicted to chocolate desserts, ordered a gargantuan portion. I ordered coffee. Watching Jack gorge himself on that fabulous dessert, smacking his lips with every turn of the spoon, made me furious. I yanked the spoon out of his hand. "I just want a taste," I bellowed. Suddenly, as though in a dream, a waiter appeared with a double portion of trifle and placed it in front of me. Jack smiled. Apparently, after he had been served his portion, he quietly excused himself, pretending to go to the men's room and had instructed the waiter to bring me that double portion. Smart guy, Jack. It was ambrosia. Like Jack, I licked the plate clean, determined not to feel guilty about it. I promised myself that I would avoid all rich food on the flight to Russia. I needn't have worried.

The Aeroflot flight to Leningrad was strictly a no-frills flight. There were no complimentary glasses of vodka, no caviar canapes, no trays of Zakuska, the famous Russian appetizers, no sampling of blini and sour cream. There was no food or drink served, except hard candy. Odd choice, I thought.

After trekking halfway around the world, we finally arrived in Russia. We were taken to the Hotel Leningrad, a relatively new, luxury tourist hotel. With great fanfare, I was shown to my room. It was the size of a utility closet, made to order for midgets and other small people, like the Lilliputians who inhabit the imaginary land of Lilliput in Jonathan Swift's *Gulliver's Travels*. The Lilliputians were six inches tall. But for an oversized, overenergized American actor with an insomnia problem and a heavy work load and who was planning a fairly lengthy stay, a room that looked like the YMCA was definitely not for me. A comfortable suite—which is what I expected—was what I wanted. But there were no suites available, I was told by the Russian concierge. "Nyet, nyet." No, no—it's their favorite word. Unwilling to take "Nyet" for an answer—I said quietly, "Get me everybody." People who know me know that when I'm in an unhappy situation and I say, "Get me everybody," I mean *everybody*—producers, directors, business managers. Everybody connected with the production.

Paul Radin, the production manager, a dear and patient man, in charge of those pesky little things—like kvetching actors—was sympathetic. "Look," he said, "there are no suites right now. The hotel is booked solid. It's the weekend," he said. "The place is teeming with tourists, especially from Finland. They come for the vodka. It's the best vodka in the world." "Great," I thought, "I don't even drink. Neither does Jack." "A suite will be ready on Monday and you can have that," Paul said.

For three miserable nights I slept in that cramped room with my feet hanging three feet off the end of the bed. I hit my head on the wall, scraped my fingers across the floor everytime I turned over, and was bruised everywhere. On Monday, I moved out of there to a suite with two rooms and a river view. I was overjoyed. It was my only truly happy moment during the whole Russian experience.

I knew the first day of shooting, we were doomed.

We began what I thought was going to be my favorite scene in the film.

In their quest for the bluebird, Tytyl and Mytyl and their loyal humanoid friends arrive at the Palace of Night. There, in a huge room, behind a monumental door that glides open as if by magic, is a garden of ineffable beauty bathed in nocturnal light. It is the Garden of Dreams. For me, it was like reaching the Land of Oz. In this ethereal wonder, an innumerable array of bluebirds hover perpetually, illuminated by the stars and planets, shimmering and fluttering among the moonbeams. Thinking they have found the bluebird of happiness, everybody is delirious, chasing after the birds, collecting and gathering armfuls of bluebirds to bring back to the Fairy Berylune.

While the scene was beautifully written, it was a nightmare to shoot. In addition to the ordinary technical problems, we now had a flock of freewheeling bluebirds to add to our technical nightmare. The bluebirds were actually trained pigeons, painted powder blue. Completely unmanageable, some broke rank and were seen flying past the commissary window. Others dizzily smashed into the eye of the camera, completely obscuring the shot. To get them to hover around us, bits and pieces of bird feed were planted in our costumes and on our heads. Catching a sniff of the bits of food stashed away in our clothing, those powder blue pigeons descended on us with unerring instinct, like birds of prey. With their strong short beaks, they pecked at the food, nipping hard at my flesh. Cornered by a flock of pigeons—who whirled madly, landing and taking off, making a loud clapping wing noise as they gathered speed for the takeoff, fluttering and hovering in the air, unceasingly flapping their wings with each turn, finally swooping down on me for another nip—I was paralyzed with fear. They landed everywhere at the same time: they landed on my head, on my shoulders, on my arms, perching wherever it was convenient and comfortable and pecking at each new spot. They pecked right through my shaggy costume, drawing blood. Underneath my costume, I could feel a slow trickle of blood. It was like the final moment in Hitchcock's horror movie, *The Birds,* when the killer birds, once tame and friendly to man, attack the Brenner house for the final kill.

More difficult to cope with was the pigeons' personal habits. They are not toilet trained. Shooting a tender scene with 500 pigeons flying overhead was messy. All around me I could hear George screaming, "Cut, cut." Most of the time was spent cleaning up after the pigeons. We never did get that scene right.

Carl Kress, who won an Academy Award for his editing of *The Towering Inferno,* was losing his mind trying to edit on a 1921 moviola. Eventually, he quit. Elizabeth Taylor arrived with 102° fever. Len Film Studios, where most of the shooting was done, was cold and cavernous, impossible to heat. There was only one toilet for the entire company. In her gorgeous Light costume, Elizabeth had to wait in line with the rest of us. Cicely Tyson, a vegetarian forced to live on cabbage leaves, was suffering from malnutrition. In the winter, there are no vegetables in Russia. The few that crop up are sold at extortion prices. On one trip to the market, Cicely paid twenty dollars for one carrot and ten dollars for a cucumber. She was headed for bankruptcy.

Another problem was that there was no way I could diet in Russia. After sampling the food the first weekend I was there, I knew I was in trouble. The hotel food was inedible, and there was very little to buy at the markets. My first meal at the hotel was chicken Kiev, a relatively simple dish, I thought. It was awful. It was unlike any chicken Kiev I have ever had before; the color bothered me more than anything. It was mortuary gray. I later learned that all Russian chicken is gray. Once Ava Gardner's maid, Emme, prepared a delectable Southern fried chicken for the company. When we asked her how she did it, she told us she had marinated the chicken in vinegar for three days. She had no tricks for improving breakfast. Eggs were generally cooked with lard; sausages looked like the country sausages called Weisswurst. There's no meat in them at all; just pure cream-colored fat. I get ill just thinking about it even now.

There was a buffet bar on each floor with slightly different menus. To break the monotony of the long hours, we used to play musical buffets, comparing menus, which consisted mostly of a variety of tasteless pastries.

I discovered the black bread and butter which is the best in the world, and lived on that for three weeks. I gained seventeen pounds. I was frantic and put in a call to Gerry Musante. "What's wrong?" he said. "Listen," I said, "I got a problem here. There's nothing to eat in Russia and I've already gained seventeen pounds." "How can that be?" he said, convinced I was overreacting as I have a tendency to do. (Also the connection wasn't the greatest.) But, after hearing me out, he understood. "But there must be something to eat in Russia. There has to be. There are eggs there, aren't there?"

"Yes."

"What about the egg whites. You could make egg white omelets."

"On what?"

"There must be something there to cook on," he said. "Find

it. If the dairy products are good, what about cottage cheese? You can make cottage cheese omelets."

He's right, I thought. Of course, eggs. Terrific guy, my diet guru. Clever man, that Gerry Musante. It was worth the $999.00 telephone call for that advice. The dairy products in Russia are the best in the world. They just are—the ice creams, the butter, the cream, the yogurt (not low-fat yogurt, it is the richest, creamiest, fattest yogurt in the world and the most delicious). It's what keeps the Georgians living until age 110, according to the yogurt commercials.

But on reflection, eating eggs was good for a short-term solution, but it was not a good long-term plan. If I continued to live on black bread and butter, I thought, what chance did I have? Four months is 120 days. If I had already gained seventeen pounds in fourteen days; that means I would probably gain 90 pounds in four months. I was desperate. I wanted out. I had to get out of Russia while I could still fit in an Aeroflot plane. After all, they're not 747s.

One night in George Cukor's suite, we decided something had to be done about the food. George said, "Does anybody here cook?"

Jack piped up, "Jimmy's a terrific cook."

George said, "What do you need?"

"Something to cook on," I said, "like a stove."

"That would help," Jack said.

"What else could you use?"

"What have you got?"

"An electric frying pan?" He smiled.

"What do I cook in it? And where will I get the food?"

"I'll give you time off from the movie to go shopping."

I could see it coming. My part would get smaller and my job as a cook would get larger. In no time at all George Cukor's bathroom was converted into a kitchen. With George's electric frying pan—that marvelous invention of American technology—and a few extra utensils we rustled up, I started cooking in. Again, I became the company cook.

We foraged daily for food. Prices were exorbitant. With Russian inflation, a head of lettuce cost five dollars. Four tomatoes cost ten dollars. The price of meat, when you could find it, was astronomical. There were none of the Russian delicacies we expected to find. Although I looked hard, there was never any Beluga caviar around. I stopped looking when I learned that the very best caviar is exported. There was plenty of the salty, gooey pressed variety, but the best Beluga was back at Zabar's Delicatessen in New York City.

After a while—because finding food in the local markets was always such a hassle—George used his clout and arranged to have food shipped regularly from Fortnum and Mason, the Zabar's of London. We ordered hams and chickens and crabmeat and many other staples. Once we even had Fortnum and Mason raspberries. The company nearly went crazy.

It was an airlift maneuver that worked like a charm—when it worked. Sometimes shipments were late or didn't arrive at all. Sometimes they sat in customs and spoiled. But generally they reached us. We waited for the Fortnum and Mason shipments like prisoners of war waiting for mail. As the packages began to trickle in, we began to dine in style.

When the English "care" packages arrived, I did the best I could, making ham casseroles, meatloaf, brisket of beef, veal cutlet, tuna casserole, veal stew, beef stew, and chicken curry. Fortnum and Mason saved the day. Long live Fortnum and Mason.

Whenever we could, we would escape. Whenever we could maneuver it or whenever there seemed to be a logical break in the schedule, Jack, Cicely Tyson, her secretary, Susan Siem, and I would fly away, if we could get exit visas. Getting exit visas took considerable will power and perseverance. There was almost no way of cracking the Russian bureaucracy. Getting into Russia was easy. Getting out was impossible. But despite the Russian obstinacy, we persisted and in time we were able to make regular junkets to Helsinki or Copenhagen or Stockholm.

On the first trip to Helsinki, which took eleven hours by train, we were almost blinded by the sun. It was the first sunlight we had seen in months. People were smiling. There was food everywhere. There were flower stalls with fresh, unwilted flowers. I mentioned that to Ava Gardner when we got back. At the sight of a banana, Cicely almost broke down. We went wild. We bought fruits and cheeses and meats and caviar. It was the first of several food orgies we would make while we fought the Russians over exit visas. As Cicely said, "It was like Robinson Crusoe arriving in civilization after being shipwrecked for twenty years." Those Scandinavian junkets saved our lives. The high point of these culinary excursions was a smorgasbord lunch at the Operakelleron Smorgasbord, a four-star restaurant in Stockholm, the equal of Maxim's in Paris both in price and quality.

When we returned to Russia, we were told that Elizabeth Taylor was in a London hospital with a severe case of amoebic dysentery, an acute and sometimes fatal intestinal disease which she had contracted from ice cubes, possibly while searching for a substitute for her favorite Jack Daniel's on the rocks.

Obviously, the Leningrad drinking water—at that time the color of mud—was infested with deadly little amoebas. Only after I left Russia did I learn that it was also contaminated by a less insidious parasite known as Giardia lamblia, a microscopic organism that causes the cosmopolitan traveler's diarrhea, carbon copy of the familiar tourista and Montezuma's revenge. Then, I understood why the cast and crew had suffered a rash of intestinal disorders, including the various stomach disorders from the food. Everybody had been sick.

After waiting four days for a visa, Elizabeth—who was deathly ill according to unconfirmed reports—finally made it to a London hospital where she was under the care of her personal physician. As she convalesced in a suite in the Dorchester Hotel, she even lost 17 pounds. I envied her.

While Elizabeth fiddled, Leningrad burned. Maeterlinck's fairy tale was turning into a disaster movie. Everything had gone wrong and as rumors circulated that *The Blue Bird* might have to shut down because of Elizabeth Taylor's illness, the cast and crew—despairing over the interminable delays and the deplorable conditions—began to take flight, like an army routed in battle.

For a week I had been working on a sequence called "The Palace of Luxury," a gluttonous banquet scene overflowing with fabulous foods. Gazing in wonder at the dazzling array of meats, my character, Dog, salivating, exclaimed, "And such game! And sausages and legs of lamb and calf's liver!" There is nothing nicer and lovelier in the world than liver, except that the prop liver looked so sickening I didn't touch it. After shooting for a whole week, I was informed I had been suspended the whole time. It was crazy.

In his penetrating book *Valentines & Vitriol* (a collection of celebrity profiles) Rex Reed—journalist, author, critic, and sometime actor—wrote firsthand about *The Blue Bird*. He described the chaos:

On the night before I'm to leave, all hell breaks loose. The cast learns by telegram they have been on suspension for the past week. All salaries have been suspended. All this time, they have been reporting to the studio daily. Cicely Tyson and Jimmy Coco finally get their agents on the phone at 6 a.m. They are informed Eddie Lewis has just told them everything is fine and George Cukor is rehearsing the musical numbers. Elizabeth Taylor will be back on the set Tuesday. "How can this be when she has just checked into a hospital in London?" yells Coco with something resembling delirium tremens. "Everyone is leaving Leningrad. What songs? What dances? How can you be on suspension if you've been reporting for work? We're dealing with a mental case."

On Friday night, the cast had a meeting to decide what to do. Tempers flared, mothers were in tears. Will the rooms be reserved if they leave? Who will pay for overweight luggage? How much luggage should they pack? Who will pay for the transportation? Will the film be resumed after the hiatus? Ava Gardner ventured forth from her Garboesque sanctum sanctorum long enough to hear the wails and the cries of gloom and doom. She had been a lady long enough. She punched the production manager, John Palmer, in the nose. Throughout the hotel, you could hear that Cinemascope and stereophonic sound voice booming: "I will not be quiet! I will not behave! Get me outta this town, get me outta this picture. I want my visa and I want my passport and I'm getting the hell outta here *tonight*!"

SATURDAY. My week ends in glorious Leningrad. Members of the *The Blue Bird* company sit around in various stages of suicidal despair on pieces of luggage strewn throughout the lobby, waiting for passports that might never arrive. As the baffled, unhappy cast prepares to depart at their own expense for places unknown, wondering if the *The Blue Bird* will ever fly again . . .

Officially suspended, we packed furiously, threw everything into a car and headed for the airport.

For all the ballyhoo about detente-cultural exchange, *The Blue Bird* was essentially a big business deal, an opportunity for both the Soviets and the Americans to make a killing as well as to make movie history. Fox had the distribution rights, the Russians had something else. Despite the commercial side of things, however, it was a rare opportunity for them to combine creative talents, no small thing either. It was, after all, the first Soviet-American coproduction ever. For Edward Lewis, who engineered the whole deal, it was a big coup. It looked like a sure thing—an American cast that included Elizabeth Taylor, Ava Gardner, Jane Fonda, and Cicely Tyson; top Russian performers like Boris Godunov; the direction of the legendary George Cukor—still the project misfired. Elizabeth never made her $2,000,000. Several times during the early days of filming I asked to be released from the film but George wouldn't do it. I think he liked my cooking too much.

For me personally it was a real letdown. Like everybody else, I had envisaged another *Wizard of Oz*. Like Dorothy and her anthropomorphized friends, we dreamed of traveling on another yellow brick road. *The Blue Bird* was going to be another film classic. What it was was an abortive effort at film making by two monolithic, lumbering giants who couldn't get it off the ground. It was an unhappy experience. As I watched it go down the drain, I was saddened. After all, I had my eye on a rainbow.

At rock bottom, I think it was a matter of temperament and different methods of working. The Russians are slow and methodical. Americans are fast and maybe glib—I don't know. To us—unfortunately, perhaps—time is money. Such a philosophy is too ingrained to be changed overnight. We're a computer society. We're fast. We're quick. We do things in a hurry. Sometimes that doesn't always work to our best advantage. We have a tendency to cut too many corners. We can self-destruct. But that's the way things are. That is not to say that people in two different tempos cannot pool their talents and create something wonderful. It just didn't happen that time, that's all.

Aboard a friendly Finnair flight, first to Helsinki, later to Stockholm, we left Leningrad for an extended Scandinavian holiday, uncertain about the production schedule. It was a last-minute decision. There was a good possibility we would spend most of the time in Sweden, as close as possible to the famous Operakelleron, the world's greatest smorgasbord restaurant. Maybe I would just move in.

But on the flight to Stockholm, I turned to Jack and said, "Why don't we just go home?" Once Cicely Tyson had gone AWOL. After five serene days in Hollywood, she returned without causing a ripple. "Listen," she explained later, "I went to California to regain my sanity." She brought back a Ouija board, Mille Bornes, Probe, Monopoly, a bicycle, peanut butter cookies and a Lhasa Apso puppy. Cicely has never been known to travel light.

We boarded Scandinavian Airlines bound for New York. On April 30, at 3:40 p.m., we touched down at Kennedy Airport. We were home. For good. But I didn't know it then.

Although I should have felt ebullient about my New York holiday, I was still troubled and annoyed by the whole Russian experience, angry about having gained seventeen pounds on black bread and butter, and concerned about a sporadic chest and abdominal pain that lingered for several weeks in Leningrad. It puzzled me. Frankly, because of the emotional strain (frustration and tension), I assumed it was psychosomatic.

Since I was home in New York, I consulted my personal physician, Dr. Michael Bruno, who had me admitted into Lenox Hill Hospital for a complete examination. I was due for a checkup anyway. Generally I was in good health, except for occasional hypertension, so I was startled to find that I had, of all things, gallstones.

The doctors recommended surgery. That was not what I had in mind for a New York holiday. But when they explained the possible serious complications of the disease, among them cancer of the gall bladder, I panicked and decided to go ahead with the surgery.

"Jimmy, before surgery, you really should lose some weight," Dr. Bruno said.

"Really, Doctor. How much?"

"About thirty pounds. Do you think you can do it? You're over 250, and it's difficult to cut through that much . . ." he paused, searching for the right word.

"Fat?" I interjected.

"Yes. It's too risky. Can you lose the weight?"

"Of course," I said, snapping my pudgy fingers. "Just like that."

Of course, that was pure bravado on my part. I really wasn't so sure.

Faced with surgery, I knew I'd be unable to return to Russia to finish *The Blue Bird*. My agent immediately told Edward Lewis, the American producer, that I would have to leave. Lewis tried to juggle my scenes to keep me in the film but when he was informed about the length of time involved to lose the weight, to have the surgery, and to convalesce, he reluctantly agreed to replace me.

After all my incessant bitching, when I was officially out of the film, something I'd prayed for daily during those dreary months in Leningrad, I felt somehow heartsick about having to leave it. I had never had to leave a job before, and now I was full of an actor's anxiety about where the next job would come from.

Actors are funny people. They scream and holler and rant and rave. They're unruly and chaotic, muddled and confused, ambivalent about most things and unsure about the rest. It's the constant deprivation. Being chronically unemployed warps the psyche and rattles the brain. The unemployment rate is always between 80 and 85 percent. An actor earns an average of five thousand dollars annually. That's about two cents an hour or $1.50 a day. Messenger boys are better off. They get a lot of fresh air and they get to stop off for a pizza. For whatever reasons, if an actor loses a part, as I did in *The Blue Bird*, it's like losing a lover. It breaks your heart.

I decided to lose the thirty pounds in Durham. With the

DRC staff preparing the meals, and weighing and measuring calories, I wouldn't have to think or do anything. All I would have to do is show up at the dining room, eat, and run. It was a routine I enjoyed. I liked the order, the discipline, the feeling of control. Away from the madness of the Big Apple I could find a peaceful solitary spot under a magnolia tree, daydreaming as I ticked off the ugly pounds and entered the numbers in my diary.

The DRC diet, of course, still worked like a charm—in Durham. At home, it was another matter. Obviously still on a diet treadmill, I returned to the diet clinic over and over, over a period of years as my weight fluctuated. I could lose, but I couldn't maintain.

Apprehensive about the operation, I concentrated on losing the weight without pondering the whys and wherefores of weight reduction. The thirty pounds seemed to drop off more quickly than usual. When you're dieting for the sake of appearance, time seems to drag; but time seems to whiz by when you're dieting to prepare for surgery. Before long it was time for the event. I lost the weight that was required. I had no more excuses. I had to face it.

The next thing I knew I was back in Lenox Hill in the recovery room. The night before the operation, I remember lying in my room being prepared for the morning operation. My body had to be shaved. The orderly who was prepping me said, "What are you going in for?" I said, "A gallstone operation." Without flinching, he said, "Oh, is that a tough one. Boy, what pain." I said, "They told me there would be a little discomfort. I was told it would only be a little discomfort."

"They always say it's a little discomfort. Believe me you're going to feel pain."

He paused and I said, "Would you please finish shaving and leave me alone? I obviously have a day of pain ahead of me, and I need rest!"

As I gradually regained consciousness in the recovery room, which must have been 32°, a radio was blaring loud rock music. Nurses were loudly calling my name, verbally jolting me into consciousness. In addition to being absolutely numb from the cold, I was famished and began chewing on something that just happened to be in my mouth. I believed that a compassionate nurse had put some food in my mouth knowing I would be ravenous when I regained consciousness. I realized later that they had put a wet washcloth in my mouth, probably to keep me from biting my tongue and injuring myself as I came to. Never knock eating a wet washcloth until you've tried it.

While I was lying there, hungry and cold, chewing on the rag, I thought, "Oh God, no. I can't start eating fattening hospital food just after returning from the weight reduction clinic."

Routinely, after returning from Durham, I would follow my structured regime for a while, but for some reason I would gradually slip back into my old eating habits. To avoid slipping into bad habits again, I asked to be put on a diet of a thousand calories a day for the week that I was in the hospital. On a thousand calorie diet, I would continue losing, not as rapidly as on seven hundred calories, but I would continue losing. It was an inspiration.

As a memento, Dr. Howard Kesseler, the senior surgeon at Lenox Hill who performed the surgery, presented me with a stone. It is a large, oval-shaped, gray-brown stone about 1½ inches in its greatest dimension. It looked like it belonged to somebody's rock collection. I still have it. It's in my memorabilia collection, displayed in a glass box in my bedroom.

As a compulsive collector with a passion for the past, I've collected movie memorabilia for years, such as old movie magazines and autographed photographs of the movie stars of the 1930s and 1940s. During my youth when movie stars made personal appearances, I would hang around the big hotels and the movie theaters, sometimes standing around for hours outside the old Capitol Theater or the Roxy on Broadway, waiting to get their autographs. The jewels of my Shirley Temple collection are a rare cereal bowl and pitcher made of blue glass, adorned with Shirley's autographed picture. On the cereal bowl Shirley says, "Hello, everybody." And it's signed, "Shirley Temple." I get goose pimples every time I look at it.

I also collect Daily Dime Banks. One is dated 1929 and pictures Popeye with his bulging muscles and corncob pipe. It is my prize possession. Another depicts that daredevil

Superman about to take off on another exploit. The banks
work like a cash register. As a dime is inserted, they display
the date and the amount. I must have about a dozen of
them.

Of course, I'm still a sucker for Mickey Mouse items. I
have a very rare Pluto-shaped clock in mint condition. Pluto's
eyes roll and his tongue goes in and out. I have always
understood that clock. You see, Pluto is salivating over his
dinner and his eyes are looking down at his dish and his
tongue goes in and out. To me, it's priceless. I would never
sell it or any of my collection. I collect for my own pleasure.
I'm not an investor.

In addition to my treasured collections, which are displayed in my living room, I have a closetful of worthless junk
which I've scavenged from the streets. One of my best finds
was a shadeless base of a signed Tiffany lamp. Another is an
extinct NBC logo that I picked up in an ashcan outside the
NBC studios. It's a peacock made of chicken wire with three
feathers missing. I have no use for any of these things, but I
can't bring myself to throw any of them away.

As a passionate collector caught up in the current American craze for the past, I even cherish my own gallstone—I
can't even get rid of that. Who knows, a hundred years from
now, old gallstones may be very valuable. I think I'll hold on
to it—unless it disintegrates and turns into dust. Maybe
then I'll just save the dust. Whenever I get moody and
depressed, I go into my bedroom and rub my gallstone box
and, like Aladdin's lamp, out comes a genie and dispels my
unhappy feelings.

On that low calorie diet in the hospital, I lost an additional
seven pounds. Before leaving the hospital I was down to a
svelte 218 pounds, for me almost an ideal weight. I was in
good spirits. Luckily I had two terrific offers for new produc-
tions scheduled to begin in the fall. One was Neil Simon's
Murder by Death, a satire of detective fiction. The other was
a television comedy series called *The Dumplings*. Needless
to say, I was so elated, I wanted to telephone for a pizza. I
caught myself just in time.

I was anxious to get back to work, so while I convalesced
I studied the Simon script. At other times, I watched the
tube and entertained friends who always arrived with cheerful-

looking boxes of nuts and candy or Italian pastries. "You've been sick," they would say. "You need to get your strength back." I never argued.

Somehow, during those months, I managed for the most part to maintain my svelte hospital weight. I had seen the *Murder by Death* costume sketches and had even had several fittings. I knew I had to maintain my weight for my character, Milo Perrier, the fastidious Belgian detective. The elegant tailored suits and the color-coordinated hand-made silk shirts, designed by Ann Roth, were extremely form-fitting. There was no room for expansion. In addition to the stylish wardrobe, Perrier sported an ostentatious gold watch and fob that rested conspicuously on his paunch. His appearance also featured a marcelled toupee and a large waxed mustache to match. I liked the Perrier look and wanted to look my best. I was afraid that if I were to gain an ounce, I would burst right out of those elegant clothes.

But I still was in good shape, though I did put on two or three extra pounds; I guess I must have weakened when one of my friends came in with a box of chocolates. I told myself that I could easily take off those couple of pounds in California. That was another canard. Through trial and error, I know that losing weight in California is like coming in on a wing and a prayer. Time to start praying. California, here I come.

Whenever I was in Hollywood doing a movie or a television show, the likelihood I'd stay structured was as remote as my winning the Mr. America contest. The production schedule is so unstructured and grueling and insane that there's no way of maintaining structured eating habits. The hours are interminable. On the set from dawn until dusk, exhausted and groggy after a sixteen hour shift, I'm in no mood to start pushing a shopping cart at the supermarket. I want to grab a fast bite and get quickly to bed. The next morning's call comes very early.

There's always plenty of food on the set. And while there's a good deal of snacking out of boredom, (waiting around for the scenes to be set up, and so on) more significant is the anxiety eating. I do a lot of it. Whenever I'm doing a new scene, I begin to get nervous and tense and slightly paranoid, too. I'd start worrying about everything and I'd grab a cheese Danish. Is the scene going to work? Will I flub my lines? Will I get it on the first take? Being conscious of 120 company members eyeing me during rehearsals only increases my anxiety. What will they think? What will the other actors think of me? Who'll get the last cheese Danish? As the underlying anxiety mounts, I head straight for the snack table, picking on anything.

Even the makeup person coming to retouch the actor's wilting face brings not only powder and paint but also refreshments of chocolate drink or coconut cake. It's hard to resist that. And then there's always the buffet table that looks as if a delicatessen had literally been moved whole onto the set, with a spread of bagels and cream cheese and nuts and danish and pretzels and peanuts and peanut butter and cookies and candies replenished daily. There's no end to that table. As a special treat occasionally, a stagehand's wife will bake something special, and a mammoth strawberry shortcake can materialize without warning and disappear the same way; or someone else might make a vat of veal and peppers.

On top of the regular all-day snacking, there are regularly scheduled lunch and dinner breaks during which the cast goes to restaurants not known for calorie-conscious meals. I couldn't discipline myself to stay behind preparing a diet meal in my trailer.

Mexican food is very popular in California. The informality and the sangria, the refried beans and enchiladas, seem to be a favorite with cast and crew. Of course, I suppose I could have shown some discipline and just nibbled on the lettuce on top of the tacos but somehow my mouth always closed in on the taco itself and before I knew it I had swallowed it. Once swallowed the damage is done.

Compounding the problem are the frantic California weekends. Instead of being a time for unwinding, weekends became a mad flurry of socializing with old friends. An entire social life was crammed into those 48 hours of intensive wining and dining, including a mad round of cocktail parties, dinners, and new restaurants. There were never-ending brunches which usually began with avocado dips and every other kind of dip imaginable, each of which piled on more and more calories. Working on the West Coast is an eating marathon.

As I settled in the plane for the long flight to Los Angeles the "fasten your seat belt" sign flashed on and so did the light in my head. In the words of Sancho Panza, Don Quixote's aphoristic sidekick, "Forewarned is forearmed." This time I would be disciplined and structured. I would not succumb to the California pitfalls: *No noshing on the set. No catch-as-catch-can meals. No weekend binges.* This time I would be strong—very, very strong. I hoped. I settled back and opened my script.

Murder by Death is the story of an eccentric millionaire who invites the world's five greatest detectives to a dinner and a murder. The whole thing is a hoax, of course, but as in any good murder mystery, the hoax is not revealed until the end.

In my opening scene, Perrier is munching on a chocolate bar. He petulantly berates his chauffeur for bringing a chocolate bar *without* nuts. I wondered if I could get a stand-in for the chocolate bar.

In the awesome cast were Eileen Brennan, Peter Falk, Maggie Smith, the late David Niven, Alec Guinness, Nancy Walker, the late Peter Sellers, Estelle Winwood, Elsa Lanchester and Truman Capote in his movie debut. Gathered together for the initial reading of the Simon script, the ensemble of famous players seem to be in awe of each other and are a little uptight. After champagne and caviar everybody loosened up and began to feel more comfortable. I know I did.

Except for Eileen Brennan and Nancy Walker, I had never worked with any of the other cast members; it was exciting getting to know them.

Peter Falk was health-conscious; he kept a handy treadmill parked outside his dressing room trailer. Periodically, Peter would be out there working out on it. He was calorie-conscious as well; he had fresh fruit delivered daily to the set. Instead of nibbling on all those fattening foods, Peter would snack on the fresh fruit. He was a model of discipline and self-control, and he worked at keeping in shape. Even for a character actor, physical appearance is an important part of his stock-in-trade. I hoped I could emulate Peter and thereby maintain my weight.

David Niven looked as if he had been born trim and dapper and debonair. Blessed with a quick wit and a nimble tongue, he probably quipped at birth, "Don't bother to look, I'm a boy." After a long and successful Hollywood career, he still looked like a Hardy Amies fashion plate. Tall and very thin, he was perfect for the parody of Nick Charles, the William Powell character in *The Thin Man*, a role for which I could never be physically right. I once asked him, "Don't you ever put on any weight?"

"If I do put on a pound or two," he answered, "I can usually work it off at a hard game of tennis or walking around the lot; chatting with old friends along the way helps too. One can walk five miles around the Burbank lot. Maybe it's just my metabolism." ("A pound or two," I thought. I wanted to hit him.)

I envied David Niven. Why wasn't I born with the right metabolism? There's a great mystique about metabolism. People argue about it constantly. Some say there are people in this world who never have to worry about gaining weight and attribute it to their metabolism. Apparently David Niven is one of the privileged few who is able to eat anything without gaining weight.

Johnny Carson is another of these lucky people. Johnny's weight has never fluctuated in the ten years since I first appeared on the *Tonight* show. I can remember thinking one time, "His waist is as big as my thigh." At the Palm—a favorite actor's restaurant in Los Angeles—I have seen him devour a huge lobster, lavishly served with butter sauce, fried onions, baked potato, and creamed vegetable with all the trimmings, knowing that he wouldn't put on an ounce. If I ate the same meal, I would put on seven pounds before I got home.

Maggie Smith and David Niven were both tall and very thin and, according to Vincent Canby's review in the *New York Times*, "looked as if they had invented the dry martini." I cannot think of a better description.

I remember Maggie at lunch one day staring at her plate. "What's wrong?" I asked. "Isn't that what you ordered?" She said, "I'm always astonished at the portions Americans serve. In England, we serve small portions. Look at the size of this steak. It's gigantic." Not to me. It looked like a normal-sized steak to me. No matter what she was served, Maggie always ate only half of it. I wondered if it were the portions or if she was really dieting and didn't let on. I never did find out. But let's give her the benefit of the doubt.

At 94, Estelle Winwood, the English character actress who recently celebrated her one hundredth birthday, is an anachronism. I once asked her, "How do you do it?"

"How do I do what?" she said.

"How do you keep in such terrific health?"

"Oh, that's easy," she said. "I smoke four packs a day, I drink, I play bridge every night. I also eat anything I like and I sleep four good hours a night."

While I can't recommend this regime to anyone, it's certainly awe-inspiring. As the doddering invalid-nurse confined to a wheelchair, she was always letter-perfect. Like an astronaut floating in outer space, she was weightless.

If Sir Alec Guinness ever had a weight problem, nobody had the courage to ask him. How can anybody ask the Force of *Star Wars*, "Were you ever a fat kid?"

But looking around me I must say truthfully that the entire cast of *Murder by Death* was a knockout.

At first, I had no problem keeping my weight down. I stayed away from snack foods as I planned. Whenever I was tense or anxious or felt a little hungry I'd go over to the fruit bowl and eat a banana or a pineapple wedge or pick on a strawberry—thanks to Peter. At other times, I would try to prepare diet meals in my trailer.

Gradually, as I began socializing more with the rest of the company and joining them in restaurants, I could feel myself weakening.

One eventful day, David, who had discovered "an incredible new Italian restaurant" invited Maggie and me to lunch. Reluctant at first, knowing how dangerous Italian food can be for me, I almost said "no." But after thinking it over for twenty seconds, I decided, "why not? I can always have a shrimp cocktail and a piece of fruit—not my idea of ambrosia, but safe! Anyway, it's better than eating alone in my dressing-room trailer, a victim of my own dietmania." So having neatly resolved the problem, I said "yes."

David, Maggie and I had become fast friends. We enjoyed hearing David's stories, and Maggie and I were crazy about Scrabble. Together we spent many long hours with the lettered tile.

As we broke for lunch that day, we started out for David's "incredible new Italian restaurant" which was about a twenty-minute drive from the studio. Finally there, I could see, beyond the restaurant's revolving door, an uncluttered dining room and crisp, clean white tablecloths. There were no corny murals of Venetian gondolas or volcanoes erupting in the background, only a bronze replica of Romulus and Remus being suckled by a she-wolf. So the restaurant was Roman. They say, "When in Rome, do as the Romans do." Well, this was one Roman who wasn't. I was sticking to shrimp cocktail.

As the waiter showed us to our table, my eyes lighted on the dessert cart which was uncomfortably near our table. There were the usual Sicilian cannoli, popular the world over, it seems to me; Zuppa Inglese, a distant cousin of that splendid English dessert, "trifle," a custardy dessert made with day-old bread, the more mundane rum cake (which I suspect is really a bastardization of something else), and a bowl of whole pears baked in wine. None of it moved me. So far, so good! Then, I spotted a scrumptious-looking cheese cake on the lower tier of the cart, oozing with glistening buttery goodness on the top crust. That began to move me. Suddenly I realized that David must have asked me a question. When I turned to the table, he and Maggie were staring at me. Finally David said, "Well what do you think, Jimmy?" Fortunately, just as I was about to bluff an answer, I was saved by the waiter who came to take our order.

All ears, Maggie and I listened as David entertained us with his famous San Simeon stories about William Randolph Hearst and Marion Davies. While David gave us the inside story about that aerie in the sky, Maggie and I munched on breadsticks and warm Italian bread. The bread kept reminding me of Giordano's, that Bronx bakery that made the world's best Italian bread or so I thought when I was ten.

As I reached for the last breadstick, the waiter arrived with our pasta. Ambrosia. In the familiar scenario that followed, this is what happened: Maggie ate half, David ate nothing, and I was waiting for seconds. What can I tell you? It's a sickness. But instead of pasta seconds, I had a large piece of that delicious looking cheese cake. It was worth the sacrifice. Finally, surfeited and well-fed, we left "Romulus and Remus," and waddled back to the Studio for another long afternoon session.

Try as I might after that, staying structured was pure hell. I knew intuitively that in a matter of hours maybe, I would break the California oath again. Damn it! History was repeating itself.

If I started that routine, my elegant Perrier costumes would no longer be elegant. They would be bursting at the seams. "OK," I said. "I did it. I'm guilty. Back to the diet tomorrow." I felt better. I knew I wasn't going to have any trouble. I was wrong. Staying away from the snack foods became harder and harder. Resisting was pure hell. Despite my good intentions, I gave up trying to prepare diet meals in my trailer. And frankly, I couldn't look at another piece of fruit. This is going to be even tougher than I thought.

And, indeed, invited again to David's "incredible new Italian restaurant," I didn't think twice about accepting. Without a qualm, I ordered spaghetti carbonara with extra cheese. For dessert—a large piece of Italian cheese cake. I was a goner.

I will never forget the day Maggie and I were playing Scrabble in her dressing room. I dropped one of my tiles. "That's a blank," Maggie said. "Lucky you." As I bent to get it, I heard the humiliating ripping sound of my pants splitting. I have a long history of that. It started when I was ten. Fat and fortyish, it was still happening.

Maggie, usually a model of English decorum, burst into a fit of laughter. "Maggie, stop laughing," I said, "get me some help. Call the wardrobe lady. Call somebody. They're almost ready for our scene. I can't go on looking like this."

As if on cue, the voice of director Robert Moore boomed over the public address system. "Ready for Maggie and Jimmy. Please get them out here."

"Please get them out here," I screamed. Maggie was convulsed with laughter. Grabbing her by the shoulders I said, "Did you hear what they said, Maggie? 'Get them out here.' What am I going to do?"

Suddenly Maggie—like the efficient Jean Brodie—snapped to attention. "Don't worry, darling," she said. "I'm always prepared for any emergency." As she reached into her purse, pulling out a small sewing kit, she spun me around bodily and said, "March." I thought, "She *is* Jean Brodie." I marched. Maggie marched behind me onto the set, sewing up my pants. "We better go over our lines, darling," she said. And we did. We reached the set on time, word perfect, and my pants were sewn so expertly that it looked as if it were the work of a professional seamstress.

I have always worshipped Maggie, but from that day, I was her adoring slave. She had won an Academy Award for *The Prime of Miss Jean Brodie.* I would gladly have presented her with another for being the most quick-witted, resourceful, unflappable, lovable woman of the year.

When Maggie's needle and thread was now put away, no one would ever have known that those pants had split in the first place.

As the film drew to a close, I had regained almost all the weight I had lost. There was no way of disguising it. I had done it again.

At the wrap party—a farewell party given at the conclusion of a film—I had a final fling with California-style eating. The *Murder by Death* party, catered by Chasen's, one of California's best and most popular restaurants, featured all of Chasen's favorite dishes including the famous Chasen's chili. There is a story that the legendary Elizabeth Taylor, a chili zealot, has Chasen's chili shipped to her wherever she may be. If this is true, that's quite an endorsement for a bowl of chili.

In addition to the chili, the Chasen menu included barbecued chicken dripping in succulent sauces, wonderfully fattening honey spareribs, a variety of breads, potatoes, vegetables, exotic cheeses, crackers, and rich desserts—none of it low-calorie, of course. But, as I was going to hell in a handcart that night, I gorged myself on everything.

As the orchestra played and people danced and embraced in the spirit of camaraderie, a barrage of colored balloons was released. As a thousand balloons floated up to the ceiling, so did my weight. Devastated over having broken my word to myself, I felt like a monumental failure. But there was no time for self-recriminations. I had another show to do.

The new NBC television comedy series, *The Dumplings*, was written and produced by Don Nicholl, Michael Ross and Bernie West, under the supervision of Norman Lear, the maverick mastermind of *All in the Family*. Obviously, the part of Joe Dumpling was another fattie. While I felt miserable about the weight, my new producers were doing handsprings. In fact, had I allowed it, they would have stuffed me like a foie gras goose, fattening me up another thirty or forty pounds. "Keep it up," they cheered, "you look great." Even my costumes were designed to look loose and baggy to accentuate my weight. Actually, being fat was physically good for the part. It was just not good for me, for my ego, my self-esteem or my health. Type casting is a terrible thing.

Based on a Canadian comic strip by Fred Lucky, a jovial, chubby, cartoonist who was an ideal model for his own funny characters, *The Dumplings* is the story of Joe and Angela, a fat middle aged couple who run a small New York luncheonette. Still ardently in love after fifteen years of marriage, Joe and Angela, reminiscing with a customer, recall how they met at a friend's party. Joe remembers spotting Angela at the buffet table. "There she was taking two portions of everything. I said to myself, 'That's my kind of woman!' So I picked up a plate and followed right behind her." It was love at first sight. To Joe and Angela, the fat protagonists, love is all. Money doesn't count. Aggression is an ugly word, and food is love. History was repeating itself.

While I desperately wanted a hit series, I was in a quandary about *The Dumplings*. Almost 250 pounds again, I physically filled the bill, but emotionally, I was in a dilemma. On the one hand, I was dying to do the series; on the other, I dreaded having to be fat for it. If *The Dumplings* were a hit (statistically, a new television show is always a long shot), I might be fat forever. Like most people, I wanted it both ways. I wanted to be a thin man playing a fat part in a big fat successful television series—fat chance, I thought with my erratic eating habits, maniacal binges and another food-loving character part. Was I destined to play only fat character parts? As I wrestled with the problem, an unexpected solution fell into my lap.

After unsuccessfully auditioning a rehearsal hall full of fat actresses for the role of Angela, Joe's adoring wife, the producers—in a typical show biz about-face—cast Geraldine Brooks, a warm attractive actress who was an ideal Angela except for her size. She was a size eight. Apparently, though, being slim was no obstacle. The producers solved that problem with padding. As Angela, Geraldine wore a styrofoam bodysuit that made her look like a size sixteen.

A light bulb went off in my head. If Geraldine could be padded, why couldn't I? No matter how much I'd lose, I could always be padded. With padding, I could lose weight and go on playing Joe Dumpling forever. What an idea. The marvels and miracles of show business.

As we began filming the first episode, hoping to make television history, finally relaxed about playing the part, I settled in for what I hoped would be a long run.

After thirteen weeks, the show was cancelled. The famous Nielson ratings did us in again. History was repeating itself, I thought, as I angrily bit into a juicy cheese Danish.

At the wrap party (a farewell party given at the close of a show), held in the set-luncheonette, we ate and drank and cried bucketsful. Actors are sentimental people. Farewells are always sad. Several of us were friends from other shows. Marcia Rodd, my sister-in-law in the series, had co-starred with me in "The Last of the Red Hot Lovers," the Neil Simon comedy that gave me my big break. Also in the series was George Furth, actor and author, whose musical *Company* had been successfully produced on Broadway. We had been in several shows together. Someday, we might all be reunited in another show. Sadly, Geraldine Brooks, a new friend, died the following year after a long struggle with cancer.

Depressed over the failure of the series I started on a merry mirthless marathon eating binge that took almost a year to run its' course. When I'm binging, I go berserk. Obsessed with food, I eat voraciously and ceaselessly, stuffing my pockets with candies and other sweets, and carry them around with me wherever I go, buy cookies by the pound, ice cream by the gallon, and nuts by the basket. In a frenzy of eating, I'll cook up a pot of spaghetti at two in the morning improvising a sauce with anything handy, a can of tuna fish, chili peppers or just garlic and oil with or without a touch of basil. And if necessary with nothing at all, just the plain pasta will do. Or in a pinch I can always order a Chinese banquet from my favorite corner Szechuan restaurant. They deliver food piping hot in eight minutes to my apartment and their telephone number is indelibly fixed in my mind. I can dial-a-meal in two seconds flat, ordering by memory one from column A and from column B. And if the eight minutes seems too long a wait for my Chinese feast, I can always pop a slice of frozen pizza into my toaster-oven. It only takes two minutes to heat up. When nobody's around, I squirrel things in secret places. Stashed away in the fourth drawer under my clean socks are bound to be three bags of a chocolate something. Since I know where the booty is buried, all I have to do is reach inside a sock and violá, out comes a Mr. Goodbar.

After almost 25 years, I was still on a schizophrenic treadmill. How long would these rampaging binges continue? How could I stop them for good. "My God," I thought, "when was the first time I had asked myself that question?" Sobered by the question, I still did not have an answer.

Reading the *Village Voice* over breakfast, I came across a crude ad for a small workshop production of a play called *The Transfiguration of Benno Blimpie*. The ad was a drawing of a fat man eating a huge hero sandwich while standing by a refrigerator.

For some inexplicable reason, I became curious about the play. Maybe it was just that hero sandwich in the ad. Perhaps it was that actors are always scouting for vehicles and good properties (show-biz talk for good plays, and great parts as rare as a flawless diamond).

So I trekked uptown to a little out-of-the-way theater on the West Side that appeared to be a converted grocery store. I caught a performance of *The Transfiguration of Benno Blimpie*; my friend Robert Drivas was right. *Benno Blimpie* was a searing, daring, sensational play by a young, undiscovered playwright named Albert Innaurato. It was my turn to call Robert Drivas. "Remember that play you told me about some time ago? About that 535-pound man that was eating himself to death?" To which Bobby answered, "When you hung up on me?" "Yeah, that's the one," I answered. "Well, what about it?" "Well, I just saw it and you're right. It is terrific. I'm aching to do it. We have got to do this play. Of course, you've got to direct it. Let's find a producer."

Benno was not considered commercial by major uptown producers because it was only a one-act play and also had strong language and explicit sex scenes involving a thirteen-year-old girl. We contacted Adela Holzer, a major investor in the rock musical *Hair* and the producer of several Terrence McNally plays. After reading the play, she said, "I don't know how commercial this play is going to be. The language is so strong. The sex scenes are very explicit. Well, then again, it might be a big hit after all. Let's do it." She decided to take a chance on it and a limited four-week engagement was scheduled at the Astor Place Theater.

Not just another fat character part, Benno was the part of a life and, in many ways, a mirror-image of myself. I felt an intuitive empathy with the character. Since I am essentially thought of as a comedic actor, the play was also a rare opportunity to do a heavy dramatic role and hopefully a chance to personally score in a bravura performance. All in all, with the excitement of discovering an unknown new talent in Albert Innaurato, the production tingled with theatrical promise.

Even at my heaviest, I could not approximate Benno's weight so that I had to be padded for the part. I had fantasized about being padded for a part. Now, the wish was gratified. When I first looked at myself in my dressing room mirror, padded and in costume as Benno Blimpie, I was shocked and frightened by the image. By a trick of theatrical magic, I had been transformed into a grotesque 500 pound man. I suddenly saw what I could become. It was terrifying. Transfixed I was unable to take my eyes from that awful possibility in the mirror. When the stage manager walked in, asking if I wanted anything, I automatically said, "Yes, a ham and cheese with lots of mayo and a chocolate milkshake." Thinking back, I am appalled that I could have ordered food while looking at that hideous creature in the mirror.

On a raised platform, sitting in a tiny chair obscured by his bulk, surrounded by the foods that he eats throughout the play, Benno methodically acts out a ritual of self-destruction. As the play opens, Benno is happily licking an ice cream cone as the audience is tittering. Facing the crowd, the character says, "I am Benno—I am eating myself to death." The audience stops tittering.

As Benno unfolds his sordid story, he recalls his deprived childhood and solitude of an estranged and hostile family. The family includes a grandfather whose perverted encounters with a precocious adolescent are symbolically expressed as she nibbles on a chicken leg. The girl impulsively murders Benno's beloved grandfather. Lured into a darkened (secluded) schoolyard by a gang of neighborhood toughs, Benno is sodomized and brutally beaten. As they stuff bits of broken glass and dirt into his mouth, Benno is left lying on the ground, threatened with severe reprisals if he informs on his aggressors. It is this cruel incident in the character's unhappy life that is finally the true "Transfiguration of Benno Blimpie."

While I never expected Benno to be a cinch, I never anticipated the problems I encountered either. Confident about the play's success, I should have been on cloud nine. Instead, straight through the rehearsal period and all through the run of the play, I was unduly edgy and tense, at times, almost trembling with anxiety. I couldn't make it out. At first, I attributed the feelings to the normal show business pressures of doing a new show and having to face the unpredictable New York critics again. But it didn't work that way.

From the beginning, as I worked on the part, analyzing and probing for the underlying causes of the character's bizarre behavior, I sensed it was something more than just pre-opening night jitters. Opening night was still weeks away. In retrospect, what did happen, I think, was that as I began searching for the historical connections between my own history of obesity and that of the character, I unconsciously unleashed, largely unresolved, anxiety-provoking conflicts that dovetailed with Benno's. It knocked me for a loop. Caught in an emotional bind with my own character, I slipped in and out of shifting moods of anxiety and depression, rage and fatigue, exacerbated by a compulsive, self-destructive craving for food that we both shared.

There were other problems, too. Since eating was the crux of the character's pathology, I had to stuff myself on fattening foods at every performance. On a steady diet of Benno-type foods, I also had to be prepared for the consequences: a catastrophic weight increase. At first I tried substituting dietetic-like foods, such as Weight-Watchers Apple Chips instead of potato chips, frozen yogurt instead of ice cream and (white?) marshmallows instead of chocolate? (Marshmallows have fewer calories than chocolate some-body had reported. Look in the calorie chart in the back of this book for the answer).

Unfortunately, eating dietetic foods just didn't work for me. No morbidly obese character like Benno Blimpie was going to bother with a dietetic food. Nor was I. It violated my sense of truth. I had to have the real thing—no substitutes, no fakes—Without them, I couldn't believe in the character I was portraying. (Or was that just an infantile subterfuge?) Actually, the added weight didn't bother me at first. Pro-tected by my styrofoam suit, I felt safe from the world's prying eyes. I could hide behind my Benno-disguise without the extra weight ever showing. That, at least, was a blessing.

While I could weather the emotional storms of playing Benno, the physical was more trying. After a while, I actu-ally began feeling physically ill from the combined off-stage, on-stage eating. One thing led to another. Hypertension, that family bugaboo, began plaguing me again as it always does when I'm out of control. It's like a bad penny. It always turns up. I even started worrying about my cholesterol, something I rarely do. My cholesterol is the most stable thing in my life. What really gave me a start, though, was a shortness of breath. I had never had that before. Barely able to walk the short distance of five or six blocks from my home to the theater, I had to stop two or three times to catch my breath. If that was the case, I was finished in the theater. There is no place in the theater for a breathless actor.

While I could still joke about it, I didn't like the feeling of having trouble on stage. That bothered me. I didn't like feeling I might have an anxiety attack on stage or worse still, a heart attack. That really scared the hell out of me.

For the first time in my life, the excess weight was affecting my ability to work. That was very unsettling. The stage is my life. That is all I know how to do. Without that, what would I do? Or if I'm so exhausted after a performance I practically have to crawl off stage, who's going to hire me? Once, I even thought I was actually having a nervous break-down on stage. Frankly, I didn't know what was happening to me. It was all a mess. Like Settenbrini, Thomas Mann's ailing character in "The Magic Mountain," I thought, is it time for me to retire to a high mountain top sanitarium and wait for the end? I wasn't ready for that. Mercifully, I thought, it's not a long run. If I could only hold out till the end of the run, then I'd see what to do. I don't give up easily.

While my styrofoam suit was a blessing in disguise, the compulsive need to imitate my character on stage and off was a curse! Driven by inner demons beyond my control, after every performance I would race home and instead of unwinding before bedtime with a simple nightcap, I would race home and raid the refrigerator. Stripped of my camou-flage clothing and safely hidden in the privacy of my home, like a mirror-image of Benno, I would stuff myself almost to the point of bursting. Despite the obvious health hazards, I repeated the scene like a nightly ritual. What was this play doing to me, I thought? Why was I so angry? Whom did I hate? On whom was I trying to avenge myself? Without answers to those painful questions, I repeated the pattern again and again and again. Like Benno, I felt vulnerable and exposed, ripped to shreds, and bone-weary in mind and body. How often had I felt like an object of derision and scorn? How many times had I experienced his humiliation and shame? How often had I been terrified and depressed. How often had I felt like a weakling and a loser? How many times had I wanted to die?

For me, Benno was not just another part. It was a transcendental experience. It was a catharsis. It was self-confrontation. It was a smash. The reviews were sensational. The actors scored. Bobby was lauded for his direction and like Rocky Balboa, Sylvester Stallone's urban folk-hero who beat all the odds, Albert Innaurato was lionized as the playwright of the season and James Coco was "rediscovered." In the words of Mel Gussow, a drama critic for *The New York Times,* "James Coco gives the performance of a lifetime." *Benno* was the most memorable theatrical experience of my life. It nearly killed me.

One night, after a performance, as I was cooling off in my dressing room, Bea Arthur, a dear friend who had come to see the show, visited me backstage. Obviously moved by the performance, but perhaps not wanting to appear maudlin, she assumed her well-known garrulous Maude stance, saying gruffly, "Well, you made me cry out there. Are you happy? Thanks for a miserable night!" After embracing and kissing and gossiping together about mutual California friends like two happy magpies, she finally said, "Okay. Enough talk. Get out of your padding and let's go for a drink."

"Bea," I said (stunned for a second) "I'm not wearing any padding. It's over there, hanging on the costume rack." Embarrassed by the faux paus, she quickly countered, "Oh, I didn't mean that. I meant take off your bathrobe. You know me. I'm as blind as a bat." Despite the valiant attempt at covering up the blunder, I knew what she meant. "My God," I thought, "if Bea thinks I'm wearing padding, so must everybody else. Can't people tell when I'm wearing padding and when I'm not? Do I look as if I weigh 535 pounds?!"

Later, sipping a drink with Bea at a nearby theater restaurant, my head was spinning. I kept hearing those words over and over again in my head. "Get out of your padding and let's go for a drink." Well, Bea's friendly Freudian slip did the trick. The next morning, I yanked out my scale (hidden from view for the run of the play). As soon as I stepped on the scale, I knew what Bea was talking about. Again, I was almost at my all-time high: 305 pounds. In gratitude for making me realize so graphically that self-improvement was definitely necessary, I sent Bea a lovely bouquet of spring flowers.

Within days, after the successful run of *Benno,* I was on a flight to Durham, North Carolina. My obesity was now a major health threat. It was affecting my ability to perform, I was in deep trouble. I meant business.

5. Success at Last: Showing Off with Carson

When I returned to Durham this time, I was fighting mad. I had been on the Rehab Diet for years, and there was obviously something wrong with it. I had developed a nice lilting Southern cadence to my speech from several trips to North Carolina, but I was still having difficulty controlling my weight at home and on the road. If this costly regimen worked only in Durham, then it was just another gimmick diet. It was a fake. Despite my frustration and rage, I felt compelled to give it one last try—and to have it out with Gerry Musante.

Dr. Musante was no longer associated with Duke; he had opened Structure House, his own weight-control center in Durham. Since I wanted to continue with Musante, at least through this final confrontation, I changed programs.

Unlike the hospital setting of the Dietary Rehabilitation Clinic, with its cafeteria-style eating arrangements, Structure House is set up in a comfortable homelike large house nestled in among graceful magnolias and towering elms in a quiet, congenial residential area of the city. For me, it was a thoroughly pleasant change from the laboratory atmosphere of hypodermic needles and blood tests and white-coated medics at the Rehabilitation Clinic.

That institutional setting and the cafeteria-style eating atmosphere had been practically my only gripes about the excellent DRC. Personally, I don't like standing in a long cafeteria line inching my way up to a counter holding on to a plastic serving tray. Furthermore, the Rehab Center dining room was adjacent to a student cafeteria that served nondiet meals. The sights and sounds and smells of sizzling cheeseburgers and french fries always left me disgruntled and irritable while I collected and ate a skimpy-looking diet serving. At Structure House there is a dining room with tablecloths, table service, and an occasional candlelight dinner. I like the amenities of a gracious table even when dieting.

As soon as I settled into this new scene I cornered Dr. Musante for what my scenario billed as the showdown.

"Now, listen," I told him. "Something is wrong. I can't go on this way. Your diet does not work. It's a fake."

I waited. He said nothing.

"Besides that, it's costing me a fortune! You know how many times I've been here?"

I waited again. Nothing.

"Sure, it works in Durham. Sure, I'm always thrilled after I have a spectacular weight loss. But what happens when I leave here? I start putting the weight back on. Will you explain that to me?

Silence.

"I'm telling you each time I leave I regain weight. How many times am I supposed to come back here? It's making me crazy. Am I supposed to move to Durham and find work in the theater here?" I noticed my voice rising as if I were on stage.

Unruffled, Dr. Musante listened intently. He swirled his iced tea and finally said, "OK. Let's discuss it. I think it's time too.

"For years, you've been taking jaunts to the clinic as if it were a resort. Sometimes you've been frantic to get into shape for a television special or guest appearance with Johnny Carson. Am I right?"

Now it was my turn to say nothing and to try to appear unruffled.

"You've always been a model patient here. You stay structured. You keep your diary. You weigh in religiously each morning. I've watched you take off all your rings and your shoes and strip down to your shorts before getting on the scale. You even take off your glasses and sometimes I'm not sure whether you're seeing the beam because you're afraid to weigh with your glasses. You've even taken off your glasses and called *me* over because you can't see the beam.

"But what happens when you go home? You told me that that last role—that Benno something—exhausted you. Frightened by your high blood pressure and cholesterol levels you come running back here, enraged and out of control. You're heavier than you've been in years and riddled with guilt. Now you attack the diet and imply that the Clinic is after your money. The diet couldn't work with a person who wasn't ready to work.

"I have patients who, after years of struggling with psychological problems, are still caught up in early pathology, unable to effect the necessary changes for desired results. Unless a person is ready for change, *it* won't work because that person is not going to make it work.

"If a person has had a weight problem for a long time, he's not going to get rid of it in a short period of time. It's unrealistic to think that after a few weeks on a diet program, the problem will disappear forever. It takes time."

"A few weeks? I've been coming here for years."

"Yes, you have, but a few weeks at a time. And in those few weeks you want all the answers. There are no quick answers. This is a step-by-step process. With the appropriate steps, a person can ultimately be able to control his weight.

"Structure House patients often have serious physical and emotional problems. Many of them are diet dropouts who have struggled unsuccessfully for years with other diet methods. Some are already experiencing obesity-related illnesses such as hypertension and diabetes. I'm talking about people with exogenous obesity. People who are overweight from overeating, not from known or unknown medical causes. Eighty percent of obesity problems are food-related. They are not from malfunctioning thyroid glands, for example, or from other physical causes as people would sometimes like to believe."

"I never thought of that. Maybe it's my glands."

"Your glands are just fine.

"Having failed repeatedly," he continued, "patients are self-deprecating, and blame themselves harshly for the lack of success, attributing diet failures to character defects.

Generally bewildered, misinformed, with a lack of understanding of the overall process of losing weight, they don't know how to approach the problem of losing and controlling weight.

"The same questions come up again and again. Why can't *I* succeed? Why do *I* have this problem? Why do *I* have the tendency to overeat? Why is food such an overwhelming part of my life?"

I wish I had a nickel for everytime I asked those questions. I'd never have to do another soap opera.

I like soap operas.

"Ultimately, a patient must realize that obesity is essentially a behavioral problem and only by dealing with behavioral and psychological causes will that person succeed in permanently losing and controlling weight."

"Well, if I've been doing all the right things," I answered, "this shouldn't apply to me. You said so yourself, I'm doing all the right things. The diet hasn't worked for me."

"The diet hasn't worked for you because you haven't been ready."

"What do you mean, I haven't been ready? Every time I come here I'm ready."

"Jimmy, you are unwilling or unable to deal with the underlying causes for your overeating. You have focused almost exclusively on the diet itself. While occasionally you have paid lip service to behavior modification and other parts of the program, you have not been really seriously interested in the entire process. You know very little about nutrition and you flit in and out of group sessions. When did you attend your last lecture here?"

"I don't remember," I answered.

"Without an understanding of your behavior patterns and eating habits which cause your overeating, you will never be able to successfully control your weight."

"What the hell am I supposed to do? Do you think I come here for a vacation? Do you think I love it here that much? It's not that I don't like you. I think you're a swell person. Next time you and Rita come to New York, let's go out. Fine, but I'm sick to death of coming here. Give it to me in layman's terms. What do I have to do?"

"If you're ready to probe and find answers to the fundamental questions all patients have to ask themselves at some point, it will work. Why is food so important to you? What part does it play in your life? How did it get to be so important in your life? These are the things you have to begin to seriously ask yourself."

"I have asked myself these questions. I have also come up with some pretty dull answers."

Sipping his tea, he stared at me for a while. I lit up another cigarette.

"Approach it as if it were a role, as if you were analyzing a character in a play, trying to find out the playwright's intention or, as you always say—the motivation of the character. Haven't I frequently heard you say time and time again 'I have to analyze my part, I have to delve into the history of my character.' Well, find out what makes you tick. Find out *why* you overeat. *When* you overeat. How much you overeat and what practical steps you can begin with to change your eating habits."

"Easy for you to say, Doc."

"I once asked you what question you were most frequently asked by your adoring public."

"Yes."

"Well, what was your answer to me?"

"Oh, I know what you're talking about. 'How do you memorize all those lines?' "

"Right.

"And what's your pat reply?" he asked.

"Memorizing lines is the easiest part of acting. Anybody can memorize lines."

"Well, don't you realize that losing weight is the easiest part of the process? By reducing your caloric intake, the weight will always come off, eventually. Some people may lose more slowly than others, but it will come off. There's nothing unique about the diet. While it's low-calorie, it is basically a straightforward, prudent diet, using common, ordinary foods. There's nothing unusual, sexy, or magical about it. You're very successful with it up to a point. Maintaining and keeping the weight is the more difficult step. It's a long-term process. That won't happen overnight. It involves all the behavioral and psychological changes I've been alluding to. That's the part that takes the longest. But you've got to understand your role before you play it and to do that you must attend the lectures. You must go to the workshop classes."

"Well, I have attended the lectures. I have gone to workshop classes."

"When? How long ago was it?"

"Some of those classes are very, very long, Doc."

"Jimmy, what else have you got to do? Oh, I know what's wrong. You're afraid you're not going to have time to do all the things you like to do when you come here—going to the movies every night, antiquing and mall-hopping and taking all those side trips. Well, there's room for both."

I felt myself beginning to listen, maybe for the first time. "Go on," I said. "Where do I start?"

"With behavior modification and changing your eating habits. It's been a long time since you've thought about that. And it's a very important concept in the whole process."

"What the hell is behavior modification? I've never been sure."

"I'm glad you asked. Behavior modification is a technique, a means, a method by which we examine our own actions, our own behavior, decide why and determine why we behave the way we do, looking for ways to make changes in ourselves or in our environment so that we will behave differently. By changing your environment, you change your behavior. That's basically what it's about."

"How can I change my environment? You know what kind of business I'm in. What are you talking about?"

"For example, let's say you don't really exercise enough. Well, what do you do? Do you keep your exercise gear in the back of the closet so that everytime you want to exercise you have to take everything out of the closet or do you say, 'Let me put the gear in front of the closet or even out in the room so when I come home, I'll see it there and I'll be inclined to exercise.' It's a minor change in one's environment but that slight change can bring about a significant change in your behavior and before long you'll find yourself exercising more."

"Well, that makes sense—I guess."

"When I first introduced the concept of behavior modification at DRC, it was still largely experimental, a new concept in the treatment of obesity. Over the years it has proven itself. While I know that you may pay lip service to the concept of behavior modification, I'm not sure you've adapted it. Have you tried it at home?"

"You mean have I tried wearing a surgical mask while preparing meals? Frankly, I've always considered that ridiculous. It just doesn't work for me. That's all there is to it. As a matter of fact, it makes me laugh. It's just silly."

"Why? What's so silly about it? Why wouldn't it work? How do you know it wouldn't work? Have you tried it? It does work. It's very effective. I cannot tell you how many initially skeptical patients have later come to me and told me what an effective tool it is. And that's what it is: a tool, a technique for changing eating habits. They're skeptical at first; they have to learn from experience. Then they come back and they say 'You were right. It does work. I never realized how much food I was consuming until I started using that mask.' Not only will it keep you from nibbling while preparing meals, it will make you aware of how much food you're actually consuming."

"What about a restaurant? Am I supposed to wear a mask in a restaurant?"

"I'm not talking about restaurants. Didn't you tell me once that at mealtimes as a child, you would hang around the kitchen while your mother was preparing meals, sampling her tomato sauce or a meatball or a sausage?"

"Yes," I said, beginning to salivate.

"That's a perfect example of childhood eating patterns that carry over into adulthood. Habits we're not aware of. We have simply forgotten the historical connection. A surgical mask might help jog your memory. Now be honest. When you're preparing meals at home—say, you're on a binge—and you're making yourself pasta and meatballs, do you taste the meatballs when they're cooking?" (Long, long pause.)

"Of course I do."

"Well?"

"Well what?"

"Well, if you wore a mask, you wouldn't be able to get the meatball in your mouth."

"I bet I'd find a way."

"One patient painted her mask with lips and a beauty mark. She got a great kick out of it."

"I wouldn't."

"I told you, skeptics have come back raving about how effective it is. If a surgical mask really seems that silly to you, try something else. The point is to alter your food environment so that gradually you will change your eating habits. The mask is just a tool. Do you keep food around the house?"

"Well, of course I do."

"Why?"

"Why? What do you mean why? Suppose I get hungry in the middle of the night? What am I supposed to do?"

"With structured meals that won't happen."

"Well, how about when my friends drop in? I have to have something to serve them. I was brought up that way. After all, I'm Italian. My mother always had food in the house. There was always something to nibble on in the middle of the night. There was always food for unexpected guests. I can't suddenly change at this point in my life."

"Oh yes you can. We're talking about changing harmful eating habits. Your mother would want you to change those. After all, I'm Italian, too.

"Unless you're talking about your unconventional actor friends, nobody just drops in unexpectedly these days."

"Hold it, who said actors are unconventional?"

"Well, aren't they?"

"A prejudiced diet doctor. Just what I need."

"Well, then, they're coming to see you. They're not coming for food. Food probably doesn't mean to them what it means to you. And real friends will be supportive when you explain why you're not stocking fattening foods anymore.

"And how about shopping? Do you go to the supermarket with a thoroughly worked out shopping list? Do you know beforehand exactly what you're going to buy? Or do you just wander into the supermarket and shop on the spur of the moment without planning your menus in advance?"

"Listen, I don't know . . ."

"And how about your supermarket? Do you know every nook and cranny of it? Generally, supermarkets are designed to snare customers into impulse buying. It's almost impossible to go in for a box of Kleenex without being overwhelmed by the sights and smells of junk foods conspicuously displayed throughout the store to entice you into buying. That Twinkie sign dangling from the ceiling like a Calder mobile is a come-on for you. Don't fall into the trap of being manipulated by food merchants trying to entice you into buying junk foods."

"Nobody can make me buy anything I don't want to."

"That's what you think. How many times have you picked up a *TV Guide* because it just happens to be by the cash register?"

"Well, actually I do pick up my *TV Guide* at the cash register."

"Well, then, they know what they're doing, don't they? Do you go shopping when you're tired?"

"Yes."

"Do you go shopping when you're hungry?"

"Yes."

"After a long hard rehearsal day?"

"If I have to."

"If you go into a supermarket feeling hungry, not only will you buy out the store, but you'll eat a whole box of chocolate chip cookies before you reach the checkout counter."

"Nuts."

"Nuts?"

"I usually do that with nuts—eat a bagful before I get to the checkout counter."

"Oh?"

"Well, nuts are better than chocolate chip cookies, aren't they?"

"It's all relative. Even with your erratic schedule, there has got to be a time when you can structure in preplanned shopping. Perhaps, Sunday mornings after breakfast. Village stores are open late. They're even open on weekends. Find a convenient, comfortable time for structuring in your food shopping for the week so that you won't be tempted to fill up your shopping cart with snack foods, processed foods, and convenience foods. Or, how about shopping by phone? Don't you have a place that delivers?"

"Sure, but I like to see what I'm buying."

"With a preplanned shopping list, you'll buy only what you

need. If, for example, you decided to have three cottage cheese lunches, buy only a pint size of cottage cheese. While a quart size might be more economical, in the long run the saving isn't worth it. You'll end up eating more than you planned to."

"Well, that's probably true. I can't stand the thought of anything being left over. If there's anything left over in the refrigerator, it isn't left over for long."

"If you keep doing these things, you will gradually start altering your eating habits. Change is the important concept here: changing habit, changing attitudes toward food, lifestyle. Then you'll get your wish. You won't be coming back to Durham again.

"Clean out your kitchen when you go home this time. Get rid of the foods you don't need. Give them to your neighbors. And get rid of the M & M's stashed away in the fourth drawer under your clean socks. Word gets around."

I had to laugh at that. "Word gets around because I told you about it."

"Nutrition is another important facet of the whole dieting process: learning about foods and unlearning misconceptions. Generally, people are completely engrossed in calories, and have only a rudimentary understanding of the composition of foods and the basic concepts of nutrition. I know you can count calories. I've watched you zip through those numbers, but how much do you really know about nutrition?"

"I think I know quite a bit."

"A knowledge of the basic concepts of nutrition is essential for planning meals at home, especially in relation to weight maintenance which is what you're really hollering about today."

"I wasn't aware that I was hollering."

"Well, you were. For example, there are hidden sources of sodium in alkalizers, in laxatives, in cough medicines, and in a string of high-sodium food additives that people are ignorant about. They haven't trained themselves to read labels either. Now, I know you read the labels, don't you?"

"No."

"Why not?"

"Well, I can't see without my glasses. The print is too small."

"So carry your glasses with you."

"Well, I suppose I could."

"What do you mean, 'I suppose I could.' I carry mine."

"Well, you like to read labels, I don't. I don't have time to read labels."

"There you go again. If you don't have time to read labels, you'll always be in trouble. The labels have to tell you what it contains. Patients also have misconceptions about foods: the grandmother of one patient lived on gelatin, when she was told that gelatin was beneficial to nails and a good source of protein. It's a myth that gelatin does anything for anybody's nails. It is a poor source of protein. Another misconception: toast does not have fewer calories than plain bread. Toasted, the moisture is removed from bread so that it is lighter in weight, but has the same number of calories. Did you know that?"

"Yes, I remembered that one."

"How come?"

"Because I suddenly started to salivate at the thought of some toast smothered in butter and strawberry jam. I do, however, remember something about mineral oil. I don't remember whether it was good or bad. What was it?"

"Mineral oil is not digested by the body, and it also destroys valuable vitamins."

"Oh yes. Now I remember, I think."

"After a while, you develop a sixth sense about foods and the principle of a balanced diet. That's why one-food diets are dangerous. On a one-food diet, there's obviously no way of getting the daily requirement of the essential nutrients. Except for the banana, which is an excellent source of potassium."

"Well, I love bananas. That's one of my favorite things."

"I know."

"Often people say, 'I think I'll go on a diet. I'll just cut out potatoes, bread, and cake.' By eliminating potato, another good source of potassium, they are depriving themselves of a valuable source of vitamins and minerals. Potato is an important diet food, because it is such a rich source of minerals, and it is actually only 100 calories."

"My favorite way of making potatoes is potato shells. A potato shell is 15 calories and is loaded with potassium. I serve them to my guests. Nobody considers potato shells a diet food. They're crunchy, crispy, nutritious, and low in calories. Like bananas, it is an excellent source of potassium, and an excellent diet food."

"Well, now you're talking. When did you first find out that potatoes were so nutritious?"

"Just now. You just told me."

"You mean, this is the first time you really heard it?"

"Well, no, I always knew it in the back of my mind."

"After a while, you'll be able to recognize the trigger foods that are behavioral problems for you. For you, it might be chocolate."

"Can we please not talk about chocolate?"

"Or it might be bagels and cream cheese for someone else."

"Can we please not talk about bagels and cream cheese?"

"Or peanut butter and jelly?"

"Can we stop talking about peanut butter and jelly? Next thing you're going to do is bring up pizza and spaghetti."

"Well, ethnic foods are a big behavioral problem for most people."

Ethnic foods—that rang a bell. Ethnic foods, always a big diet problem, is the one thing I find difficult to live without.

"So since ethnic foods are always behavioral problems, and I can't live without them, I'll never be able to diet successfully. Well, we finally found the answer, didn't we, Doc. So that's it in a nutshell, isn't it?"

"Who said you have to give up ethnic foods?"

"You did."

"No, I didn't. I didn't say you can't have your pasta or eggplant parmigiana or meatballs. If it's structured into your menu planning. There's no reason why you can't have ethnic foods. Naturally, if you just ate pizza three times a day, that would be a one-food diet and you would be nutritionally deficient. I'm talking about structured meals including ethnic foods."

"Are you telling me I can have linguine and clam sauce?"

"Of course, you can. The key word is structure. Structure. If you structure it in your meals, then there's no reason why you can't have it."

"Wait a minute. Are you saying I could structure in spaghetti and pizza and still be able to diet?"

"Of course."

Structured ethnic eating. That was something I had never thought of.

"That could make all the difference. Ethnic foods have emotional associations such as mother, comfort, love, security. That's what those foods usually mean to people. That's what it certainly means to me. Giving up those foods would be very difficult."

"Food has different meanings to different people. To many people it's more than life-sustaining nourishment. Like ethnic foods for you, it's love, security, entertainment, distraction. Generally, people overeat for three main reasons: habit, boredom, and stress. That's what we have to try to understand: the antecedents of our overeating. Do you eat because you're bored?"

"Certainly not."

"Because you have nothing to do?"

"I always have something to do."

"What about those long breaks you tell me about when you're shooting a film? Hours on the set. Isn't that a little bit boring?"

"A little."

"How many times have you told me how much pressure there is in the theater? How tense and anxious you become with a new part in a play? The pressure of opening nights?"

"Well, that's true."

"The anxiety of the reviews."

"Please, let's not talk about reviews."

"How much of the overeating is job-related?"

"Now, that's important. You want to know something, Doc?"

"What?"

"I think I'm beginning to understand. Maybe for the first time."

"You want to know something, Jimmy? I think so, too. Now, why don't you go back to the hotel and go antiquing and think about what we've been talking about."

Suddenly I forgot how angry I had been when I first sat down in his office that day. He had turned the tables on me:

I didn't give him what for, he gave *me* what for. And you want to know something? I deserved it. That was a big step for me, admitting that I deserved it. Shock therapy.

After that long talk with Dr. Gerry Musante, I began to think and feel differently about the diet program. I looked at it in a completely new way. I had a lot to learn and a lot to relearn. But this time I was ready. Clearly, Dr. Musante had been right. I had been mainly concerned about the short-term gains (that is, *losses*) but hadn't actually focused before on long-term consequences and long-term changes—and weight-loss maintenance. It was time to take stock, to reevaluate, to implement the techniques and concepts of behavior modification, to examine my own lifestyle seriously and gradually to make the necessary changes.

I got right down to it. I figured I had a great deal to make up. I bought a crisp new notebook, sharpened three pencils, and got to work. For the remainder of my stay in Durham, I attended every workshop, saw all the videotapes, attended counseling sessions. I even took notes. There wasn't time for my customary daily trips to the malls and those excursions to the antique stores. I missed them, but in the end it was worth it.

I even began to turn into a sort of diet maven and slowly began to preach the gospel of the diet process. I started to lecture people, argue with them, explain, and try to educate.

One day a particularly crabby patient said "What are all these boring lectures for? Why do I have to sit here counting calories? Just give me a chart to look at. Somebody's already figured all that out. Why do I have to spend all my time in a classroom?"

It sounded like my earlier self. But now I was a convert.

"Well, you have to know what you're eating," I proclaimed. "It's the *only* way to control your food intake. Unless you understand the composition of foods and the individual calorie count, how are you going to know what and how much you are eating? If you know a banana is 90 calories, you will be able to plan a structured meal around that banana when you're at home. You can't be slipshod or imprecise about calories and nutrition or you'll constantly blow the diet. It will never work for you.

"There can be no guesswork about any of this, or it will

never work for you, either. You have to know how many calories are in a piece of pie so that you'll know that a single piece of pie is often more full of calories than a whole structured dinner."

Dr. Musante would have been proud of me.

The woman yawned and took off to see the sights. One audience I obviously didn't hold.

Not long afterward, something happened that brought the whole thing further into focus for me. Walking through the Southgate Mall, I almost collided with another dieter in my program as she was coming out of Baskin-Robbins. She was licking a colossal ice cream cone topped with chocolate sprinkles, nuts, and a dollop of hot fudge. The hot fudge sauce had congealed, forming a thin coating of chocolate around the top and the sides of the cone. It looked as if she had bought all 31 flavors. I recognized three of my own favorites: German Chocolate Cake, Baseball Nut, and Pralines 'n Cream.

Seeing me, she stammered almost inaudibly "No, no! You don't understand," punctuating each word with a gesture toward the cone.

"What don't I understand?"

Groping for words, she stared at me, holding stationary in the air the sugar cone construction that looked like an Andy Warhol pop art painting.

Still pointing a free finger at the cone, she repeated: "No, no! You don't understand!"

"Yes," I said, staring straight back.

"I haven't had any breakfast."

"Oh," I said. "Of course! Now I understand. You didn't have your ice cream cone at breakfast this morning. Just what diet program are you on?"

"No, no"—she was gesturing—"this ice cream cone is 160 calories." She smiled.

"Okay. I'll buy that. Now, how many calories are in the ice cream *in* the cone? Not to mention the sprinkles and nuts and the hot fudge?"

"No, no!" she said. "You don't understand. I'm not going to have any lunch or dinner."

"Oh," I told her. "Now everything is very clear."

She shambled away, ice cream running down her arm. Frankly, I wanted to lick it off.

Testing myself, I walked into Baskin-Robbins to check what new flavors they were featuring among their 31. Immediately I spotted Rocky Road, one of my top favorites—a chocolate ice cream filled with nuts, marshmallows, and chocolate chips. Almost tempted, I walked away, pleased that I had resisted.

Later at the hotel, just for the hell of it, I checked out the calorie count for a triple cone. A single scoop of Rocky Road by itself is 204 calories. Times 3—we're talking over 600 calories. . . .

All this talk about sweets reminds me of my friend, Jane Bergère, a Durham "buddy." Whenever she is within five feet of a candy counter, her body automatically shifts into high gear as she prepares to lunge for her favorite sweet. Holding her back is a man-sized effort. In a recurring dream, her world is a Salvadore Dali landscape with a giant box of Snickers bars into which she can reach at will. In that surrealist setting, she imagines herself dragging the box off to a secluded corner and munching voraciously while high overhead in a limpid sky, judgement and restraint lie safely out of reach. In Durham, she never has that dream.

When I got home, I cleaned out my freezer. My neighbors inherited my frozen Sara Lee cheese cake, my Baskin-Robbins Rocky Road ice cream, Jimmy Coco's Devil's Food cake, and Jane Bergère got my frozen Snickers bars.

After giving everything away, I had a feeling of loneliness and deprivation, as if something special and treasured was being taken away from me. It wasn't true deprivation, naturally, since the choice was my own. I had voluntarily determined not to have food around, to set about breaking those lifetime habits. And, as Musante pointed out frequently, if I decided that I wanted something, I could always go out and get it; nobody was tying me to a bedpost. If I suddenly wanted a stuctured—or, more likely, unstructured—Baskins-Robbins Rocky Road ice cream cone, the choice was mine. Nobody would say no. I was in control of my own destiny.

Eventually, once I had the diet program mastered in my head and understood the relationship of the different parts, I began to adapt it into what worked best for me. I began to experiment and to invent my own recipes. Some were horrendous. Some I simply had to throw away. Others were terrific, and the more I experimented the better they got. Everybody loves my veal loaf. I serve it with peppers and roasted potatoes garnished with parsley. By candlelight. It is a structured meal. *People* magazine featured it in one issue.

During the successive years of reinforcement (including some return visits to Structure House), I have learned a lot about myself, my phobias and anxieties, my hangups, stresses, my own historical reasons for overeating. A lot of things I was afraid to ask myself I asked myself. There is no magic pill. But there are answers. Mastering overweight is an ongoing process, a never-ending one. But at least I understand. As I wrestle with the stresses of creative work, relationships, chasing Maeterlinck's elusive Bluebird of Happiness, the stresses may never disappear. If they don't, I have the tools, the techniques, and the knowledge and determination to keep working at overcoming them. I will probably always have to struggle, but I will win.

I had a scheduled appearance on the *Tonight* show the day Johnny Carson announced that, after seventeen years, he was going to leave the show. It was quite a night in several respects: Word of Johnny's announced departure was top news in the papers and on the evening news shows. All hell had broken loose at NBC. With Johnny in the saddle, the *Tonight* show grossed about $115 million a year and accounted for about $23 million of annual NBC profits. Fred Silverman, then network president, who was having big troubles with low ratings anyway, was hysterical. The usually calm and reserved Fred de Cordova—the show's producer— was unnerved.

I was feeling terrific and especially looking forward to being on the Carson show that night. I had recently gotten back from Durham, where I had lost 75 pounds. After that lifetime of struggling with unsuccessful diets, I knew I had finally hit a winner. I was ready to preen a little, to show off my personal triumph. And I wanted to spread the word—to tell people that there is a way to lose weight and keep it off.

For this appearance I'd gone all out and bought myself a whole new outfit. I bought a beautiful blue blazer and a pair of Italian gray flannel slacks in a chic specialty shop on Rodeo Drive. I splurged on a Ralph Lauren shirt and an elegant polo tie. I spent a fortune on a pair of Gucci boots. I was determined to look my best.

At home, after my shopping foray, I tried on the entire outfit, relishing the stylish tailoring of the jacket, the sleek cut of the Italian pants, the soft sheen of the Gucci leatherwork in the boots. After parading back and forth in front of the mirror, testing angles, enjoying the sight, I gave one last approving glance at my new silhouette. "Boy, do I look good. Wait till they see me tonight!"

I hung everything carefully in a garment bag to be ready to grab when the NBC driver arrived to take me to the studio. That's standard procedure for most talk shows: you arrive in street clothes, then change just before going on. I placed the $300 Gucci boots carefully but prominently underneath the garment bag. When the driver arrived at the usual time I grabbed my clothes and the boots and headed for still another appearance on the *Tonight* show.

Although I've been a regular on the show for ten years, I worried about the same things I always worry about whenever I do it. Will the audience be receptive? Will they laugh? Will I bomb? Will I remember to zip up my fly? Actors never get over preperformance jitters.

At the studio there was an aura of doom, a feeling of impending disaster—a sort of just-barely-controlled hysteria. Was the show going to be canceled? Silverman had demanded that Johnny honor his contract and remain as host. Johnny had repeated in a press conference that he wanted out. Everybody seemed tense and out of sorts, dropping things, bumping into one another, nobody saying much.

Everybody was so preoccupied that hardly anybody noticed my arrival—and nobody noticed my missing 75 pounds. I practically tiptoed into my dressing room, hung up my garment bag, and began to feel miserable too. I started worrying about what was going to happen to the show, like everybody else. And remembering all the happy times on the *Tonight* show—*I* also began to feel very nostalgic. I heard the orchestra tune up and then, on the small television monitor in the dressing room, I saw Doc Severinsen "warming up" the audience with rapid-fire chatter.

In the hall outside, Richard Dawson—Johnny's guest host—paced back and forth rehearsing his opening monologue. On this of all days he was substituting for Carson for the first time. He had been ashen when I went up to him to say hello. He was probably worrying about those same things I always worry about: Would the audience be receptive? Would he get laughs? Would he bomb? Would he remember to zip up his fly? My attempts to reassure him had been no use. Dawson was a nervous wreck. I was his first guest that night, so I figured I'd better get ready. Dawson was still pacing when I passed him on my way to change after going for a light makeup.

At exactly 5:30 p.m., when the taping starts, Richard Dawson stepped out onstage and began his monologue. He gradually began to build after a sluggish start. The audience was warming up to him. He made some very funny political jokes that went over well. Before long he had hit his stride and was on his way, untroubled any longer about the Johnny situation or holding the audience. His monologue went remarkably well, I thought. The audience *was* receptive. They *did* laugh. He *didn't* bomb. He *had* remembered to zip up his fly. As I watched Dawson on the monitor I began to get out that beautiful new outfit I had prepared so painstakingly earlier. It was almost time for me to go on.

After getting into my shirt and tie, I reached for the Italian gray flannel pants I had bought on Rodeo Drive for $200. I slipped them on and they immediately dropped to my ankles. What the hell was going on? For a moment, I didn't know what had hit me. I had to be in front of the cameras in three minutes.

I suddenly realized what must have happened. I had inadvertently put the wrong pants into the garment bag at home. That was the only possible explanation. I had an old pair of gray flannels that look very similar to the ones I had bought for the show—with one big difference. The old pants were size 50, and I was now a size 38. I couldn't move. I was riveted to the spot, confounded and confused. Then, like a shot, I bolted from my dressing room and went tearing along the hall screaming for the wardrobe lady. I nearly tripped over my slipping pants in the process and could have broken a leg. Hysterical is too tame a word for what I was feeling. Panic is more like it.

The wardrobe lady heard me and came tearing down the hall to check on what had happened. She took one look at me and became hysterical herself—laughing. But wardrobe people are used to all kinds of backstage costume mishaps. Zippers get stuck, shoelaces break, seams split. So, without so much as a backward glance, the wardrobe lady took charge of this situation. She spun me around and went into action. She grabbed the seat of my pants, bunching the fabric together in big clumps, and started pinning it up. When she finished, there were five giant safety pins stuck in my pants and a very unattractive bulge sticking out.

"I feel like the Hunchback of Notre Dame," I told her. Nobody's going to even notice that I've lost all this weight, I thought.

Once she had the pants securely pinned up, she got me into my jacket and propelled me in the direction of the stage. I didn't want to go on looking like that—with that big lump protruding from my back. I wanted to go home. Start all over again. Come back another time. Come back when Johnny and NBC had resolved their contract problems and I had resolved my pants problems.

Suddenly I heard Richard Dawson's voice: "And now, ladies and gentlemen, please help me welcome my first guest, an old friend of ours, James Coco." There was no turning back. No starting over this time. I made my entrance feeling like Quasimodo.

Although I tried to be calm and composed at first, I just couldn't pull it off. No sooner had I started to sit down than something happened to me—spontaneous and unrehearsed. I turned to Richard.

"Look, I want to be honest with you. I am extremely uncomfortable —let me show the audience why."

I removed my jacket, turned my back full view to the audience for a good long look. A cameraman panned to a closeup of my rear end. It brought the house down.

When the audience finally quieted down, I told them exactly what had happened—how I had mixed up the two pairs of pants. After letting my hair down like that (in a manner of speaking), everybody—even the producers who

had been so uptight all day over the Johnny announcement—
settled down to an evening of fun.

Whenever I've been on the Carson show, I've always
leveled with the audience. Possibly that's why I have been
so regularly invited back. The audience responds to that
kind of straightforwardness, I believe. Because of that tack,
which I've taken since the very first time, I have built up a
good rapport with the TV viewers. There is, I think, a
feeling of mutual trust and respect.

The first time I was asked to do the Carson show, after
the opening of *Last of the Red Hot Lovers*—Neil Simon's
comedy about a middle-aged man having an identity crisis
(or was it a sex crisis?)—the same thing happened: I blurted
out the first thing that came into my head—spontaneously.
Friends and relatives, not to mention my agent, had advised
me how to behave, what to say, what to do, telling me to
"come on like a big Broadway star. After all, this is the
Tonight show. Millions of people will be seeing you for the
first time. Act the part!" I was so nervous that first time out
on the Carson show I could barely talk. Everybody's advice
had gone from my mind and what came out was the first
thing that had come into my head. I think it was "I'm so
nervous I think I'm going to faint." Johnny howled. After
that he was marvelous with me, immediately putting me at
ease. Carson knows instinctively how to handle people—
how to bring out the best in them. He can very deftly
change the subject if an actor is off and things are not going
well. If an actor guest is on a roll and things are going well,
he knows how to keep things rolling with his clever ad-libs
and his genius for improvising. There is a great sense of
give and take in working with Johnny Carson, and a sense of
security and know-how. You know you're working with a
real pro.

Well, that very first night, once I got started, there was
no stopping me. Before long, I went on about everything. I
talked about personal, private things people had warned me
not to talk about, like growing up in the Bronx and being so
poor we didn't have a phone. We would have to use the pay
phone in the candy store next door. That night I also talked
about my sister, who had brought me up after my mother
died, and about my father, who had remained a simple

Sicilian shoemaker. About how thrilled my father was that I was the spokesman for Drano. He would always tell his customers "Don't turn off the commercial. My son is Drano." I talked about my beloved mother, who had died when I was thirteen.

Over the years, I've told a lot of stories on the Carson show. People stop me in the streets and say, "Oh, I loved that holdup story you told on the Carson show. It was hysterical. Is it true? Did it really happen?" "And what about the story of meeting the stripper in a plane who carried her boa constrictor in her handbag?"

Well, this particular evening really took off, too. I had leveled with the audience and it had paid off again. I finally talked about Structure House. I told about the times I was so desperate I would sit in the hotel lobby in North Carolina, waiting for somebody to drop a Raisinette on the floor by mistake. I talked about that poor, desperate person who was so starved for sweets she checked herself into a hospital and sent herself a candygram every day—the doctors couldn't understand why she kept gaining weight. I talked about everything.

The response to that segment of the show was phenomenal. I was flabbergasted how many desperate people there are out there in need of help—thousands and thousands of overweight people who didn't know how to help themselves. I began to wonder if there was anything that could be done about it.

Letters and calls poured in from people everywhere, with hundreds of questions about the diet at Structure House. How did I do it? Could I keep it off? How much did the Structure House program cost? Where is Durham? Do I have to go there to lose weight? Can it be done at home? How does one start?

One letter that touched me a lot began:

Dear Mr. Coco,

I am very interested in the Structure House you mentioned on the Tonight Show. You look good after losing 75 pounds, how long did it take you to lose it?

I need some type of program to lose weight. I'm 5'2" tall and close to 500 pounds. I don't remember ever

*being thin, in fact I entered kindergarten at 110
pounds. I've been told by a number of people that my
name was mentioned on the Merv Griffin Show during one of his shows on dieting, as being the shortest
and the fattest person in the United States. It's not
something I would like to be noted for.*

*I've been in a hospital on three separate occasions
to lose weight, only to gain it all back once I was
released. I never came closer than 150 pounds over
normal weight.*

*The doctors I've been to can't find any physical
reason for me to gain weight. But they can't explain
why I gain weight on a 1000 calorie diet. When I was
in the hospital they put me on a 500 calorie diet, and
every so often I'd gain 10–15 pounds over night. The
doctors accused me of stealing food off of other patients trays, and wouldn't believe me when I told
them I wasn't. Each time I was there the same thing
happened, the doctors told me to leave the hospital
because I was defeating the purpose of being there by
stealing food.*

*I was wondering if you would send me some more
information on the Structure House. It sounds like a
very good program, and I am so tired of being fat.*

I began to wonder if there were some way to reach all
those people—a way to answer their important questions.
Unfortunately, I couldn't answer each and every call and
each and every letter personally—it would take forever.
Besides, how satisfying is a single letter? How lasting? What
can be accomplished, really, in a single phone call?

And then one day it hit me: I'm going to write a book
about it. I had found at Structure House answers to many of
those questions and been able to apply them successfully at
home. I'm going to tell people how to do it, I decided. I had
learned a few tricks. Now it was time to show them—to
spread the word. *If I can, you can.*

Part II
If I Can, You Can

6. Give Me the Structured Life

In preparation for the book, I reviewed the notes I had taken. What follows are some of the most important points necessary for fundamental menu planning and food-lifestyle change—to take weight off and keep it off.

Coco's hard-learned First Law is this: *There is no magic avenue to losing weight and keeping it off.* There is no button you can push, no machines or pills or potions that will do it for you, or even help you do it for yourself. There are no gimmicky diets or movements that will do it fast or painlessly *and* permanently. But if you're healthy and really ready, you can do it for yourself. I did.

A Healthy Lifestyle

What is a proper diet for a healthy lifestyle? Certainly not what most Americans consume—too much sugar, too much salt, too many additives—too much of everything. The American diet is probably dangerously high in cholesterol; it is certainly dangerously high in saturated fats.

Those things aside, the American diet is crammed, rammed, jammed to overflowing with unnecessary *calories*. We take in every day many more calories than our bodies use up in energy and all the processes of staying alive. What is left over is stored as body fat. That's why my diet concentrates on calories first and includes a comprehensive table of that number of calories in practically any food and drink you will ever need to know (pages 213–245). Nobody can cut down on caloric intake without knowing how many calories are in something.

My diet plan begins with a 21-day 700-calorie-a-day intake and progresses gradually to 1000 a day, then to 1200, 1500, and up to 1800 (still a losing intake), until you reach your weight goal and can finally maintain it by discovering how many calories it takes to maintain your weight.

My diet is also a balanced food program designed for real people to use or adapt in getting down to a healthy weight *for them* and then staying there. For me, for instance, 200 pounds is a healthy, manageable weight level (300 certainly wasn't!). For you it will be something different. We're dealing with sensible realities and not silver-screen fantasies.

A number of things have to change if you are going to get down to a healthy, normal weight. They include your attitude, your lifestyle, your food environment, and what and how you eat. My approach assumes that you are healthy; you can't (and usually shouldn't) attend to the task of weight control while you are physically ill or concerned about matters of health.

And, unless you are among the tiny percentage of Americans who have a genuine problem with glands or metabolism, you're overweight because you eat too much—and probably unwisely, too.

Second, *you weigh too much because you eat too much.* Your metabolism does not interfere with your being at a proper weight. You have to realize this in order to begin to know that you can indeed gain control of your weight. Metabolism will merely, from time to time, affect the rate at which you lose after you've begun to discard fat and excess flesh. Contending that some metabolic or glandular problem keeps you from losing weight and keeping it off is a copout that will keep you from making the changes necessary.

Third, *you must find the cause for your overeating.* Overeating is what we do; overweight is the result. We have to see that we're faced with an eating problem rather than a weight problem. We can't remedy the weight until we first attack the eating. We have to give attention to the reasons for this eating problem of ours, and how it developed. We then have to address the causes of our own overeating—and do some adjusting—at the same time as we adjust our own daily intake of calories for weight loss and maintenance.

This leads us back to familiar territory. Eating is far more than something most people do just to maintain life and health while we concentrate on other activities (although that's pretty much what it should be). It is very close to the top of the list of day-and-night concerns. It becomes a sort of "fork-jerk" reaction to boredom, frustration, stress of every kind, fear, and depression. And we're assaulted constantly, particularly through television, with appealing images of things to buy and eat.

We eat because of *habits* transferred from one generation to the next as well as through habits and unconscious food rituals we also build up for ourselves over the years. There's not much difference in our frames underneath it all—maybe only a ten- to fifteen-pound differential, even in people who weigh 250 to 300 pounds. The heavy-frame theory is really a diversion as far as weight loss is concerned. Much more crucial are the early childhood patterns of eating that we still hold on to, often without realizing it.

We eat, too, as a response to boredom. We eat during commercial breaks, on a dud television evening. We fill the boring voids that result perhaps from frustrations, anxieties, and disappointments. Few of us ever feel hungry. What we experience is appetite, and appetite and hunger are very different. Most often we respond to cues associated with learning to eat—times, places, circumstances. Once you learn to replace cues and put activity in the place of boredom, you're on the right track. The learned appetite pangs will decrease—and so will the sense of depression that sometimes goes along with the first stages of a decreased food intake.

We've also learned to respond to stress and tension by eating. Stress is unavoidable in modern life, but we can learn to identify the tensions and anxieties we feel and therefore cope with them better. This is a complex subject, and one for which some seriously overweight people may need to have some outside help.

Many people who have a serious weight problem—like me—have tried and tried and tried, and failed. As I did, they have followed every new regimen that came down the pike.

Many of them (like me) lost weight—and gained it back. Why didn't we succeed? Certainly not because we didn't try hard or because there was a flaw in our characters. The main reason was that the routines we followed were based on gimmicks (one-food diets, for instance), and all of them were incomplete. I have evolved a complete long-term approach to weight control that now works for me. It has continued to work for me well enough and long enough so that I am confident that it will continue to work, unlike those other fiascos. I have been able to work out my own program and stick to it without an elaborate or formal support system, although supportive family and friends like the ones I'm lucky to have are a great plus. And I still have those moments—and you will too—but I get stronger and stronger every day and am functioning very happily on my own structured, prudent diet.

And now to the nuts and bolts that will hold the Coco diet construction together sturdily.

Behavior Modification and Environment Control

The phrase sounds mildly ominous: *behavior modification*. But in dieting terms it is really a good thing and simply means interrupting problem eating habits and patterns. Breaking them, of course, implies identifying them so they can be broken. Things that can be as simple as putting away all those dishes of candy and nuts and fruit. Or throwing out junk food and calorie-crammed snacks. Or leaving the serving bowls of food in the kitchen. Breaking the nibbling-between-meals pattern. Eventually derailing the vicious cycle of overeating.

Behavior modification is really simple, I finally learned—after a mere seven years or so. It's identifying and defusing those unproductive and self-defeating eating habits, whether or not you take the time to figure out exactly how you developed them.

I had taken many notes at Durham on the behavioral approach to the problem of obesity. We discussed the nine steps of behavior modification, beginning with a restructuring of the environment. *Structure the kitchen,* the nutritionist in Durham had said. What follows are the nine steps of behavior modification based on the Structure House program.

STEP 1: RESTRUCTURING YOUR KITCHEN

1. Store foods in the kitchen, not in other rooms.
2. Eliminate snack foods from storage—particularly your behavioral problem foods.
3. Throw out any party food you save for unexpected guests.

The removal of those foods that are behavioral problems for you is crucial. A food is a behavioral problem if you can't stay away from it and it frequently appears in your unstructured eating. All rooms in the home are important. To keep food lying around in other rooms, usually sweets and foods of high carbohydrate value, can create behavior habits for children and other family members as well as yourself. *Remove it.*

The snack problem is a tricky one. The bowl of potato chips on the coffee table near your chair while you watch television, the little dish of candy on your bedside table, the little silver bowl of peanuts— they mustn't be there. We're programmed to reach for something to munch on while we read or watch television.

One thing I have changed on the calorie-snack front is this. In the theater, when I am in a show, my English dresser Harry Edwards always used to have tea waiting with two shortbread cookies when I came back to my dressing room. So I told Harry, "No more shortbread cookies. Food should be in the kitchen, and a dressing room is not a kitchen."

STEP 2: MENU PLANNING

1. Plan the meals each week in advance.
2. Write in a diary the meals planned for the week.
3. Use food group and calorie guides to plan meals.

You decide *ahead of time,* that is, you structure what you are going to eat as far ahead of time as possible. *Structure* is the key concept in the formation of new eating habits. It is similar to the skeleton of your body or the structure that holds up a tall building. But in order to structure ahead of time, you must design *menus* based upon proper nutrition and a caloric deficit. So now we have: *Plan your menu.*

Plan meals in advance, a week at a time. This eliminates indecision in the store, impulse meals, nonnutritious meals, snacking. Sit down to think about food once a week—not four or five times.

Use the calorie guide to plan your meals (but don't ignore balance for good nutrition).

List exact quantities needed on your shopping list. Make certain you include everything you need for each recipe in the week's menu plan—avoid extra trips for forgotten items.

My schedule is hectic, particularly when a play is in rehearsal or has just opened. Nevertheless, I take time even when there's a busy week ahead to decide and list what I'm going to eat for the week. When I'm in New York, if there isn't time or I don't feel strong enough to face the supermarket, I call the wonderful Jefferson Market not far away from my home and ask them to deliver what I need. (On the road and in Hollywood I also make up a weekly menu plan, even though I'm not going to be able to prepare all my own meals.) If I'm going to have a dinner party on, say, Thursday night, I'll order the proper amount of veal round or whatever for my famous veal loaf. I also cook food and freeze it in serving-size portions if I know there is a heavy schedule ahead of me. In effect, that's my way of menu planning, and it works very well for me. But I *do* plan a structured weekly menu (an example is the one on pages 157–212) and remind you that you must, too. Otherwise you'll be *really* unstructured and pretty soon you'll defeat all your goals.

STEP 3: PREPARING A SHOPPING LIST

1. List the exact quantities of each food needed, using your menu plan.

2. Group the foods according to your supermarket setup to facilitate shopping.

3. Make sure you have all foods needed for each recipe in the menu plan.

After you have meals for one week planned, you are ready to make a shopping list.

1. Go over the menus.

2. Group the items according to *areas* of your supermarket. You don't want to spend a lot of time in that store. Fifty percent of all food buying is based on impulse—that part of buying that is unplanned. So you want to make a list to use as a map in getting you through the store.

3. Be sure to write down correct *quantities* of food on your list.

STEP 4: BUYING FOOD

1. Shop on a full stomach.

2. Shop from a prepared list.

3. Spend as little time in the supermarket as possible.

Now that you have the shopping list, you are ready to be in greater control in the supermarket. But to increase that control even more, here are a few suggestions:

Shop after a meal; don't shop when you are hungry. Don't take the children if you can help it. They will frequently ask you to buy unstructured foods. Use your shopping list. In this way, you will come home with fewer items not on your list. You will avoid impulse buying. You will go through the store more quickly using your map of the store layout.

After the complete list is ready, head for the store if you're doing the shopping yourself. Get what's on that list and *get out*! Don't let yourself be tempted by that alluring little devil that keeps winking at you—Aunt Whoosiz's new ultraposh fruit cake with brandy-butter icing.

You've planned it sensibly. You've written it down. Don't blow it when you get into temptation territory. Stay as sane

and controlled inside the store as you were before you
entered it. Buy only what you planned to buy. Then make a
graceful exit as rapidly as possible.

STEP 5: STORING FOOD

1. Store foods in non-see-through containers. Use tinfoil
   instead of plastic wrap.

2. Store only foods that need to be cooked before eating.
   This makes one more step for you before practicing
   unstructured eating.

3. Store all foods out of sight—not on counter tops or
   tables.

Storing foods in a structured way means making them
less available to you, either visually or physically. Remember,
it has been found that if you have a weight problem, you
may respond to visual cues more readily than the person
without a weight problem. Therefore, you want to keep the
food out of sight. Also, you want to store the food so as to
minimize the length of time for preparation and measuring at
meal times.

Store foods in the kitchen—out of sight, not where you're
going to be looking at them every time you come into the
room. Store things in opaque containers, not clear ones.
Store only foods that need to be cooked before eating.
Make as much as possible from scratch. Run, do not walk,
away from the two-seconds package-to-table "convenience
items." Their prime convenience is to the cause of un-
needed extra calories. Store foods in the *kitchen*, not other
rooms. Get the candy dishes and filled fruit bowls out. Clear
the decks.

My living room contains what a living room should. On
the traditional coffee table—a *book*. No plates of thin-shaved
Genoa salami and pepperoni, as I have been known to leave
around in the past. No food trap is suddenly going to catch
my eye and hand. No candy on the night table. Or beside
the telephone.

No storage of snack foods—especially those that are trigger foods for you. Or foods with sentimental associations.

You don't need snack junk foods. No little goodies for unexpected guests. So I no longer keep in the house for guests food I cannot eat myself. If I give a dinner party, I serve guests what I can eat. They don't know they're eating "diet food"; I don't tell them. If there are leftovers (which I try not to have by realistic preplanning), I freeze them—it's all structured food. Or I put into the refrigerator a portion that fits into my menu for the next day and freeze the rest for other days or another party. If you plan and cook the right amount, there will be no leftovers. This is a good rule, particularly during the weight-loss phase, especially for those of us who will eat anything if it is there in the refrigerator. One habit that is important to change quickly is the compulsion to eat any leftover food because there are starving children far across the world. There are, sadly, malnourished children and adults in every country, but putting an extra 500 leftover calories into your mouth is not going to help them. Or you.

STEP 6: PREPARING FOOD

1. Wear a surgical face mask to avoid eating while preparing food.

2. Learn to measure the proper amounts needed by family members for a low-calorie high-nutrition diet.

3. Store all foods out of sight; not on counter tops or tables.

Preparing foods in a structured way means you *must know ahead of time* what the meal will consist of and what you are going to put on the table. Of course, what you decide the meal is going to be and what ends up on the table can only be made the same by measuring. You need to keep your diary particularly well during food preparation so that you can determine what your pattern of behavior is. If you are a nibbler you must interrupt that food before it gets into your mouth.

Comes the time for preparing the meal. Break that habit of lollygagging lovingly through every motion! It's one way of caressing the food you have to limit. And it leads to tasting this and that (for flavor and doneness, you tell yourself) while you are preparing the meal.

Plan and cook the right amount. Learn to measure proper amounts. Know how many calories you're putting in.

Prepare foods quickly and simply, then get out of the kitchen.

STEP 7: SERVING FOOD

1. Serve preplanned portions of food appropriate for your family.

2. Put the correct amounts on the plates before bringing it to the table.

3. Serve food in an attractive way with appealing colors and taste combinations.

Again, if food is readily available, you may eat it just because it is there. So you need to do something to keep extra food off the table when you serve. Also there are a lot of psychological cues related to food. For example, if you serve 400 calories on a typical large dinner plate, it may look like very little. Try using smaller dishes. Lastly, it is important that you keep the food handling for yourself at a minimum at this point.

Serve appropriate preplanned portions. *Do not* serve "family style." Family style means seconds. Let nondieting guests or family members get their own second helpings from the serving dishes in the kitchen.

Well, kitchen for kitchen purposes does make some sense. So does having a regular place to sit down to eat. Time was, I would walk around the house with a plate of food, eating at the kitchen counter while I answered the phone, or carrying it with me when I went to answer the doorbell. Now I do not eat standing up, moving from one room to another, watching something on television. I sit at my lovely oak dining table (which I bought twenty years ago for sixteen dollars and which must be worth a fortune now) with a proper table setting. That is important to me now.

Sitting at an attractive table with a good-looking setting, cloth napkins, matching flatware and matched plates, eating tasty and attractively served food all goes together. It's especially important psychologically, when you're dieting, to prepare attractive food and to have a good, integrated table setting. Eating should always be a pleasant experience; dieting or maintaining a weight level certainly doesn't change that.

STEP 8: EAT

1. Wait a minute.

2. Lay down utensils between mouthfuls.

3. Slow down so that your meal will last at least twenty minutes.

Waiting one minute before you eat, putting down your utensils between each mouthful and allowing at least twenty minutes for eating are all helpful. Eating slowly helps you to feel fuller. It takes some time for the message to get from your stomach to your brain that you are full. Slowing down your eating also *can make* you feel relaxed. Finger foods—foods we need to eat with our fingers—are generally fattening, so using a knife and fork for *all* eating is important. Lastly, make an effort to put *all* your food on the table: soup, main course, fruit—at the same time. Eating these separately gives you a feeling of not eating as much as when you see it all out on the table at once.

STEP 9: CLEANING UP

1. Sprinkle pepper on any leftover food. (While that's something that's done at Structure House, I do not like to spoil any food. I try not to have leftovers.)

2. Don't leave any extra food in pans or on the table but throw it out.

3. Clean up right after eating.

It is most helpful to clean up first any extra foods remaining in the pans. If necessary, sprinkle pepper on your food that is left on the plates or in the pans. This keeps the eating limited to the structured meal. Also, get your family members to clean up their own foods. Have them clean their plates, dumping leftovers into the garbage. Remember leftovers seldom find their way to another meal.

We've already mastered how to eat, and—with luck—by now it is a gracious, enjoyable minimum of twenty minutes munching.

So we've structured the kitchen. We've done our menu planning, organized a shopping list, to avoid the subtle supermarket trap. We've discussed the buying pattern: in and out. We've said it's important to store food out of sight in extreme cases—perhaps even take the light bulb out of the refrigerator. Use aluminum foil wrapping, not clear plastic. Streamline food preparation and serving. Clean up fast.

In case you don't realize it, you're on your way to mastering the nine steps for structuring the food environment at home. You've started to minimize your exposure to food. You've effected a lifestyle change!

7. Nutrition: A Drama in One Act

Everybody knows nutrition is important, but how many people can tell you why? Most people know it's a science and, unless you are a scientist, terms like hemoglobin, molecules, amino acids, tryptophan, lysine, arginine, and so on, will put you to sleep "faster than a speeding bullet."

When we got to this section of the book, it almost caused a rift in an otherwise idyllic relationship between me and my collaborator, Marion Paone. Since we have been friends for longer than either one of us cares to admit, she was the ideal person for the job. We had performed on stage together, we both have an affinity for things Italian, and we had both been to Durham together. Marion, who is 5 feet 3 inches tall, weighed in at 173 pounds the first time she went to Durham. Today, under 120 pounds, she is a true success story, having managed to keep off the weight ever since.

But when it came to the nutrition section, her mulish attitude toward facts and my cavalier attitude toward details almost caused a blistering breakup. I felt the section should be as brief and as informative as possible. She felt it should be as long as it had to be to "get in all the science."

For a spell, we were in an "I don't think we should see each other for a while" deadlock. But we soon got over that. We've been friends far too long to let a few differences of opinion come between us. We had labored long and hard over the nutrition section, trying to sound more knowledgeable than we were and knowing less than we thought. So we thought it important enough to arrange a taped interview with the Structure House nutritionist, young, vibrant, pretty Pat Andrews (who was a little pregnant at the time), pumping her for all she was worth. This is what we found out. We think you'll agree it was dramatic.

Curtain rises. The three players are seated around a coffee table in a charming Greenwich Village apartment.

MARION: Pat, what we're going to ask you may seem very rudimentary, but bear with us.

PAT: Okay.

MARION: What is nutrition? And why is it important to know about nutrition?

PAT: Nutrition is the study of nutrients, which are substances required by the body in order to function properly. You need to know about the nutrients in order to achieve proper nutrition, especially so you maintain health during weight loss. Is that clear enough?

MARION
& JIMMY: So far. Go on.

PAT: Many people attempt to lose weight by using fad diets, but fad diets don't give you enough of most of the nutrients. You end up with a deficiency of some sort. You must have all the six major nutrients in proper balance.

JIMMY: What are the six nutrients?

PAT: You mean you want me to name them?

MARION: Yes, that's what he means.

PAT: Okay. Protein, carbohydrates, fat, vitamins, minerals, and water.

JIMMY: Water is a nutrient?

PAT: Water is a nutrient. It's the one nutrient that's needed in the greatest amount every day, but each of them is required. One is not more important than another.

JIMMY: I never knew that water was a nutrient.

PAT: Well, it is.

JIMMY: It wouldn't even occur to me that water is a nutrient.

MARION: Jimmy, water is a nutrient!

PAT: They used to call calories nutrients.

JIMMY: They did?

PAT: They did, but no longer. That's because from the three primary nutrients—proteins, carbohydrates, and fat—you get calories automatically. The others—vitamins, minerals, and water—don't have any calories.

JIMMY: They have weight, of course, water has weight. But that passes through the body.

PAT: Through the system.

JIMMY: Through the system . . . and it's a nutrient!

PAT: Right.

JIMMY: Is there any truth to the theory that salt retains water in your body?

PAT: Salt does indeed cause your body to retain water. The molecule of sodium acts as a sponge in a way. It draws water and holds on to it while it's in your system. So, if you eat an excessive amount of salt, chances are you'll carry around a good bit of excessive water. When you cut your sodium intake, you lose all the extra water that's accumulated because of the presence of that sodium.

JIMMY: So you must think it necessary to be salt-free while on a diet?

PAT: No. You hear a lot of sensational headlines about sodium, because there's generally too much of it in the diet. But don't go to extremes, because you *do* need some. Just don't use salt at the table or in your cooking—

MARION: There's something else, too. People have to avoid buying canned foods, don't they?

JIMMY: Absolutely. Absolutely.

MARION: Because canned foods are heavy in salt.

PAT: Well, most are. But listen, if you do these three things, you can stay within an acceptable range of sodium intake. One, learn what the high sodium foods are. Read all labels carefully. All processed, packaged foods (the so-called "convenience foods") carry labels that give you a

	pretty good idea of sodium content. Use these foods sparingly, if at all. Two, don't add salt in cooking, and, three, don't add salt at the table. Do this and you'll end up with somewhere between 1000 and 3000 milligrams of sodium each day, which is exactly what the recommendation is.
JIMMY:	Whose recommendation is that?
PAT:	That's the recommendation of the Research Council which has basically established what requirements are for—
MARION:	—Research Council from where?
PAT:	The National Research Council, which is an arm of the National Academy of Sciences. They put out the Recommended Dietary Allowances every few years. They have established the minimum recommended allowances for each of the nutrients. Their recommendation for sodium is approximately 1000 to 3000 milligrams each day. My own feeling about it is that people who are trying to lose weight and who are counting calories really should not attempt to count milligrams of sodium unless they have a medical problem like high blood pressure, kidney disease, or a cardiovascular problem. These people have to be extremely careful. But if you're normal and healthy, sodium is a small worry.
JIMMY:	Pat, that's so clear and important.
MARION:	Are more people aware of nutrition these days, Pat?
PAT:	Yes and no. I think there's much more awareness of the importance of nutrition, but, unfortunately, most of the information people receive is misinformation, especially in diet books that emphasize one nutrient over another, like the Stillman Diet or the Atkins Diet or . . .
MARION:	But not like *Jane Brody's Nutrition Book*?
PAT:	No. Her book is not a diet book.
JIMMY:	It's quite a remarkable book, isn't it?
PAT:	It is very, very good.
MARION:	Pat, now that we know what nutrition is, what exactly do the nutrients do?

PAT: A nutrient is basically a molecule which assists the body in performing a particular function. Nutrients help the body do what it must do to survive.

MARION: Can you get too much of the nutrients?

PAT: There are certain nutrients that you can overdose on, primarily the fat-soluble vitamins: A, D, E and K, because your body doesn't rid itself of them every day. All the other vitamins are water-soluble—the eight B vitamins and vitamin C. Excesses of these vitamins are simply excreted in the urine. The fat-soluble vitamins get stored up in body fat. And if you take too much vitamin A, for instance, you could get liver damage or even liver failure.

JIMMY: Funny, most people feel you can't get enough of any vitamins.

PAT: Right. But remember that the fat-soluble vitamins (A, D, E and K) can be dangerous in so-called megadoses. And any megadoses of water-soluble vitamins will just pass out through the urine. It's unnecessary. It's expensive. It's a waste of money.

JIMMY: But what are the vitamins that are essential?

MARION: All vitamins are essential.

PAT: All vitamins are essential.

JIMMY: All vitamins are—How many vitamins are there?

PAT: Thirteen. The four fat-soluble and nine water-soluble. All of them are essential, and all of them can be gotten from food. However, it's really very difficult to get all the vitamins on a low-calorie diet.

JIMMY: So that we, who start on a 700-calorie-a-day diet, must supplement with what vitamins?

PAT: Any one-per-day capsule that includes minerals would be adequate. You do not need megadoses. And you can get generic vitamins that are less expensive than brand names.

MARION: We ought to get this very clear.

JIMMY: We know that on 700 calories, it's very hard to get the nutritional balance.

PAT: Yes.

JIMMY: Now, how do we explain that in the book?

PAT: Do it very straightforwardly by saying, "It's very difficult to get all the nutrients you need on a low-calorie diet." Period.

JIMMY: And then follow that by saying it's important to supplement your diet with a vitamin-mineral capsule.

PAT: Right.

JIMMY: However, what about when we go on our diet and graduate to a 1200-calorie day?

PAT: If you plan carefully, you won't need vitamin supplements.

JIMMY: And we *will* plan carefully, but why not take it anyway. You're not going to OD on it.

PAT: That's fine.

JIMMY: I feel instinctively that when you are used to a low intake of calories, say 700, and then you suddenly go to 1000 calories, which is still low—

PAT: Uh-huh . . .

JIMMY: I've always believed you're going to gain weight; simply because you're eating more calories than your body and your system have been used to.

PAT: Not at that level.

JIMMY: Not at that level?

PAT: No, Jimmy, not at that level.

JIMMY: But I always do, although it levels off.

PAT: Well, those extra 300 calories usually carry extra sodium—which can lead to water retention. But the fat loss is continuing the whole time and that's a real important thing to recognize. Anytime you eat fewer calories than your maintenance level you are *always* burning fat, although the scale may not reflect it because when you jump up 300 to 500 calories you might have eaten two extra slices of cheese which gave you more sodium. The next day you get on the scale, there's a half-a-pound gain, but you're still losing.

JIMMY: You're always burning fat?

PAT:	You're always burning fat on a 700-calorie diet.
JIMMY:	Even at 1200?
PAT:	Yes.
JIMMY:	So then, would it be advisable, say, to go on a diet for 21 days at 700 and shoot to 1200 calories, or should we gradually—
PAT:	It's probably wiser to gradually increase it to avoid sodium—
JIMMY:	Go to 1000, then.
PAT:	Right.
JIMMY:	So if you went on a 700-calorie-a-day diet for 21 days and, say, the following two weeks, we graduated to 1000 calories, then two weeks after that, you went to 1200 calories—
PAT:	It's probably not even necessary to go two weeks. You could do it in less.
JIMMY:	In other words, go one week on 1000, then the following week go to 1200 and then find however many calories are required to maintain your desired weight.
MARION:	What is the maintenance level of calories?
PAT:	You can arrive at that through a standard formula. If women multiply their weight times 12 and men multiply their weight by 15, that would give you approximate maintenance levels based on light physical activity.
JIMMY:	All right. I am 210 pounds . . .
PAT:	So you can eat roughly 3000 calories a day.
JIMMY:	And maintain? That's incredible.
PAT:	That's if you have light activity. Now, if you're *very* sedentary, it would be a little less than that. If you're very active, it would be a little more than that. You know, a 120-pound woman needs only 1400 or 1500 to maintain to stay at 120.
MARION:	I'm around 120. 1400 or 1500 calories a day is quite a bit.
PAT:	Well, it's a surprisingly accurate formula.
MARION:	Now, where do the 12 and 15 come from?
PAT:	From formulas that have been devised from different research groups and again, it's a ballpark

	figure. It's not going to be right on the mark for everybody.
MARION:	But what does it represent?
PAT:	It represents something called the basal metabolic rate plus light activity.
MARION:	Pat, what about protein? What is a protein?
PAT:	Protein is often called "the building block" nutrient, because it's a molecule which has the property of giving structure and form to different body parts. It is made out of smaller nitrogen-containing units called amino acids. There are 22 amino acids in all living tissue, and amino acids are simply the smallest unit in a protein. And you can make different proteins by combining different amino acids. The protein in your hair is different from the protein in your fingernails. And both of those are different from the protein in your muscles. Now your body can make all of these amino acids except nine. These nine are called essential amino acids because we can't produce them and must get them through food.
JIMMY:	And do the nine essential amino acids have names?
PAT:	Yes, they have names.
JIMMY:	Do you know what they are?
PAT:	Do you want all the names?
MARION:	Please.
JIMMY:	Do we really need to know them?
MARION:	Yes.
PAT:	The essential amino acids are methionine, threonine, tryptophan, isoleucine, leucine, lysine, histidine, valine, and phenylalanine.
MARION:	The tricky thing here is the definition of "essential"—that people understand what essential means as opposed to nonessential.
PAT:	Again, essential refers to the fact that you cannot produce them and must get them from food. It's important to know that there are some sources of protein that will give you all nine in one fell swoop. Those are the animal sources: meat, chicken, fish, milk, eggs, and cheese. If you're a vegetarian, there are some good vegetable

sources of protein like beans and nuts and legumes, but alone they don't give your body all nine. That's why vegetarians combine proteins: they eat beans and rice together. There are various combinations. Vegetarians who eat cheese, eggs, and milk are obviously better off.

JIMMY: Now, what about we who are on diets? We know beans, legumes, and nuts are good foods but high in calories. We don't have those in our diet. So, we must get them from other things—like steak, right?

PAT: That's very tricky. A lot of people believe that protein foods are less fattening than carbohydrate foods. That's completely false. Usually the protein sources are the higher calorie sources. Protein usually comes along with fat. Meat has a lot of fat in it. But potatoes don't. Potatoes, which are carbohydrate, are about 90 calories so you could have 2 whole baked potatoes for just 180 calories, but a steak weighing the same amount (say 5 ounces) even trimmed of all fat— very lean—would be 300 calories. The calories in steak will vary greatly with the amount of visible or marbled fat. Most carbohydrate sources don't have fat in them. Most protein sources do have fat in them. And fat is more than twice as high in calories than either protein or carbohydrates.

JIMMY: You mean fat is not a protein. I keep thinking fat is a protein.

PAT: No, it isn't. Just another nutrient.

JIMMY: This is where I got mixed up because I always thought of protein as fat—animal fat.

PAT: That's because they are often found in the same source.

MARION: Now, how much protein would you say—in meat—we really need to get on a daily basis?

PAT: You need the equivalent of about six ounces of meat each day for the whole day.

MARION: You do? What does equivalent mean? Does that mean a substitution like cheese and eggs and milk?

PAT: No, there's something that we go by at Structure House that most nutritionists use as a guide. It's called the "basic 4 foods guide" and if you use that then you don't have to measure out, say, grams of protein. The recommended dietary allowance for protein is about 45 grams each day, but instead of counting grams of protein, all you have to do is eat the equivalent of six ounces of meat. One ounce of meat would equal two egg whites or one egg or a half cup of beans.

JIMMY: In other words if I wanted to have three ounces of meat and one ounce of cheese or one ounce of something else as long as it totaled six ounces—

PAT: Essentially—but cheese is in a different category. Cheese is in the milk group. Cheese does give your body protein, but the recommendation is to get the required six ounces of protein from the meat group.

JIMMY: That's the first time that's been made clear to me. I always thought as long as you had a certain amount of protein daily, it doesn't matter where you get it from. Why is that? Why from the meat group?

PAT: Those are the best sources of complete proteins.

JIMMY: So what would too much protein be?

PAT: There's really no limit on protein per se. You can't really reach toxic levels unless you're unhealthy. People with kidney disease and liver disease have to limit the amount of protein they eat, but if you have a normal liver and normal kidneys, you'll just break down the excess protein and excrete all the byproducts.

JIMMY: But too much protein at one time would certainly put weight on you.

PAT: Not necessarily.

JIMMY: But if I had a two-pound steak . . .

PAT: The calories in that meat come primarily from the fat.

JIMMY: I see. I'm confusing protein with say, steak, which I know is a protein . . .

PAT: Protein source.

JIMMY: Right. Fat is another nutrient. Now, I cannot imagine, so you correct me, why fat is essential.

PAT: We need nutritional fat to create body fat, which provides both protection and insulation for the internal organs. And it is not the fat itself, but the essential fatty acids *in* the fat which are so important. There are three of these essential fatty acids.

JIMMY: What are those three?

PAT: Linoleic, arachidonic, and linolenic.

JIMMY: That's easy for you to say.

PAT: Fat is also necessary for the absorption of the fat-soluble vitamins. Remember? A, D, E, and K!

JIMMY: I remember, I remember. But the word *fat* still has such bad connotations. I mean, this is what we're all fighting against!

PAT: Well, what we are fighting against is too much of the wrong kind of fat.

MARION: Explain.

PAT: Well, you've heard the margarine commercials that ballyhoo polyunsaturated fat. That's the right kind. It contains the essential fatty acids. It comes from vegetable oils. The other kind, saturated fats, are the wrong kind. This is animal fat, and saturated fats are the ones implicated in heart disease. These are the fats that carry cholesterol.

JIMMY: Is it true that the highest cholesterol levels are in egg yolks?

PAT: Yes, but, curiously, the egg white has none. Egg white is pure protein, the standard, in fact, by which all protein is judged.

JIMMY: Isn't there a problem with eating too many egg whites?

PAT: Absolutely not; at least not if the egg whites are cooked. Too many raw egg whites can lead to a deficiency of folic acid, which is one of the B vitamins, but as soon as the egg whites are cooked this is not a problem.

JIMMY: Are we all susceptible to high cholesterol?

PAT: No one is quite sure. The body produces choles-
          terol (in the liver) and most people feel that most
          of the extra cholesterol we get from saturated
          fats, which is to say from meat, raises the choles-
          terol levels in the blood. There seems to be a
          correlation between high cholesterol and heart
          disease. However, there are people who eat lots
          of red meat and don't have high cholesterol, and
          vegetarians who eat no meat and do have high
          cholesterol, which suggests a genetic connection.
          Still, the evidence leads me to feel that you'd be
          smart to cut back on cholesterol as much as
          possible.

JIMMY: Which also cuts down calories as well.

MARION: Does that really follow?

JIMMY: Sure. For instance, if we use diet margarine
          instead of butter we get less cholesterol and
          fewer calories.

MARION: Well, yes, but we must be careful, Jimmy, to
          make the distinction between regular margarine
          and diet margarine, because some regular marga-
          rine has the same number of calories as butter.
          It may be polyunsaturated and, therefore, better
          for your heart, but it's no better for your waistline.

PAT: Fine. And most so-called diet margarine is just
          regular margarine that's been whipped up with
          air and water. You can do it with butter, too.

JIMMY: Diet butter, really?

PAT: Yes. The problem is, although it is fewer calo-
          ries per teaspoon because of the air and water,
          people tend to use more of it.

JIMMY: So what's the point?

PAT: You tell me.

MARION: Let's get back to the discussion of nutrients.
          What's next?

PAT: Carbohydrates?

MARION: Perfect. What is a carbohydrate?

PAT: Well, first I want to say that carbohydrate is my
          favorite nutrient. Carbohydrates are great food,
          the best, really, and yet they have a bad name.
          Now, to begin, there are two kinds of carbo-

hydrates: the complex and the simple. Another way of saying it is starches and sugars. There's also fiber, but we'll discuss that later. And alcohol, also.

JIMMY: Wait a minute. You mean sugar is a carbohydrate?

PAT: Yes. But there is sugar and there is sugar. You're thinking of table sugar which is just empty calories. But you know there are more calories in a tablespoon of fat than in a tablespoon of sugar.

MARION: What are the other carbohydrates besides sugar?

PAT: Other carbohydrate sources, you mean. Simply stated, everything that grows in the ground. Certain kinds of plants contain carbohydrates, protein, and fat, but all plants are primarily carbohydrate. Speaking of sugar, all carbohydrates are made up of sugar. The simple carbohydrates, the ones we *commonly* call sugars, are made up of either one or two molecules and the complex carbohydrates of many.

JIMMY: All this talk about sugar! Say, that reminds me, what *is* blood sugar?

PAT: Glucose.

MARION: What does glucose do?

PAT: A lot. Glucose is the basic fuel for most cells. In fact, your brain and nervous system generally run *only* on glucose. Your body prefers to use glucose as fuel.

JIMMY: What else can it use?

PAT: Fat and protein, but that's not good. Fat, protein, and carbohydrate all provide calories, but fats don't burn completely. The waste products from incompletely burned fats are called ketones, which in overabundance are dangerous. You don't want to use protein as the primary energy source, because nitrogen is left over when it is burned and excess nitrogen can harm the kidneys. High protein, low carbohydrate diets are dangerous. You get too much excess nitrogen, too much cholesterol from the fat that comes along with the protein, and too much ketosis.

JIMMY: I remember when I was on the Atkins diet I had

	to urinate on a stick and see how purple it became. He actually wants you in ketosis.
MARION:	That's also true of the Scarsdale diet.
PAT:	And it is dangerous. Never forget that the brain relies on glucose which is available only from carbohydrates.
JIMMY:	So we really need lots of sugar?
PAT:	You only *need* the sugar that your body frees from the complex carbohydrates it digests. The same rule that we established for salt can apply to sugar. Don't use it at the table or in cooking.
JIMMY:	What about honey? Or natural sugar?
PAT:	By natural I guess you mean unprocessed. Some honey is raw, unprocessed, whereas table sugar is processed, but it's still natural. It comes from sugar cane. And in spite of what the health food stores tell you, sugar is sugar. Honey or turbinado sugar are not more nutritious than table sugar.
JIMMY:	What about pasta? It's starch, but does it also give you sugar?
PAT:	Yes.
MARION:	You mean the body breaks down the starch molecule into sugar molecules.
PAT:	Exactly.
MARION:	What causes the starches to break down?
PAT:	Enzymes.
JIMMY:	Down in Durham there's another clinic where people go on a rice diet. Now rice is a carbohydrate, yes?
PAT:	Well, first you asked about pasta. Like so many carbohydrate sources, pasta has gotten a bad rap. Why? Because people load on fat in the form of cream sauces and butter. Now grains like rice, oats, and wheat are all excellent sources of complex carbohydrates. In combination with other complex carbohydrates, especially legumes, they also provide complete proteins; that is, proteins with all the essential amino acids.
MARION:	What about the distinction between kinds of rice?
PAT:	Basically, it's all the same rice, just differently processed. Brown rice is rice in its "natural"

form. White rice is simply rice with the brown hull "polished" off. Brown rice is more nutritious because that hull contains some B vitamins and fiber.

JIMMY: What is wild rice?

PAT: Wild rice is not a rice.

JIMMY: It's not a rice?

PAT: It's a grass.

JIMMY: It's a what?

PAT: It's a grass.

MARION: And it's not even a rice.

JIMMY: Why do they call it wild rice?

PAT: Because it looks like rice.

MARION: Potatoes?

PAT: Potatoes are great food, carbohydrate, vitamin C, fiber . . .

JIMMY: Aha! Now tell us about fiber.

MARION: Is it a nutrient?

PAT: Fiber is actually a form of carbohydrate. We lack the machinery to break it down.

MARION: What does fiber do that's beneficial?

PAT: It's beneficial in that it helps the food move through the intestines with regularity by giving the food bulk.

JIMMY: But—well, then, is cereal fiber?

PAT: Cereal contains fiber. Anything that's a plant contains fiber.

MARION: What is the nutritional value of fiber?

PAT: It has very little value because it's not broken down and it's not absorbed.

JIMMY: But it is good for our digestive system.

PAT: You should know that there is a problem with too much fiber.

JIMMY: Constipation.

PAT: Yes, too much fiber can lead to constipation so whenever you increase your fiber intake, you must also increase your liquid intake. Fiber creates bulk by absorbing water, which makes it expand. If you put in a lot of fiber and not enough liquid, you can create a blockage. Too much fiber also tends to bind up certain trace

MARION:

PAT:

MARION:

PAT:

MARION:

PAT:

JIMMY:

PAT:

JIMMY:

PAT:

MARION:

PAT:

elements. So if you have a lot of fiber you may end up deficient in things like calcium, zinc, and iron, but that's rare and not likely to happen.

Oh, Pat. You also mentioned alcohol. It's also a carbohydrate, correct?

Yes. As you know it is made from grains or fruit, like corn for bourbon or grapes for wine. Alcohol contains calories, all derived from carbohydrates that have been broken down primarily into simple sugars through distilling or fermentation. Those calories are essentially empty.

So it's not very good for you.

No, and in excess it is deadly. There is some evidence that very moderate amounts of alcohol may be healthful, but moderation is really the key word here.

We touched a moment ago on processing when we were talking about rice. There is all this talk about natural and organic. What's it all mean?

In most parts of the country "organic" means nothing. Technically, organic means "containing carbon." That is it. Health food stores sometimes use it to refer to food that has been grown without pesticides, but there is no real legal definition of the term.

So, it doesn't mean much.

It doesn't mean anything. And "natural" sometimes refers to food that has not been processed. Natural means not processed. But there's no legal definition for that either.

Then we find out that some health food stores just buy ordinary carrots, dirty them up, pass them off as organic and charge outrageous prices.

That's right.

Are health foods more healthful?

No. Although foods that are unprocessed are more healthful. But that's because processing often destroys the nutrients in food. On the other hand, so-called natural foods are no better than the unprocessed food in *any* supermarket. Chemicals have a terrible reputation, but ultimately every substance on earth has a chemical structure. For example, when you look at the molecule of vitamin A that is in that carrot and at the molecule of vitamin A that's been manufactured, they're exactly the same molecule. The body takes them apart in exactly the same way. So there's really no difference. We've all been scared away from something manufactured by man, but your body doesn't care. I feel generally good about the chemicals that are in American food. A good nutritionist knows that everything in a food is natural. The difference is processed versus unprocessed. That's where I hope you'll put your emphasis rather than bringing in the word *natural*. Because when you bring in the word natural, you associate yourself with health food people who in many cases, unfortunately, are shysters and you don't want that. What you want to promote is good nutrition. If I were you, I would avoid using the word natural altogether. Whenever you talk about foods that have the highest number of nutrients in them, bring in the words processed and unprocessed. Unprocessed foods have a higher nutritional content, often, than processed food.

JIMMY: Also, I'm going to say that I, personally, drink Tab. Marion doesn't. I also use half package of sugar substitute in my coffee. But that's entirely up to the individual.

PAT: That's great. Great.

JIMMY: I do it. I'm not afraid of it.

MARION: What would you say, Pat, would be the proper approach for a book on the subject of carbohydrates in general? How should we talk about it?

PAT: You really have a chance to separate yourself from the pack by making a statement that's different from the fad diets. I hope you'll say that carbohydrates are required and important. They should be included in a balanced meal. At every meal. The bad headlines about carbohydrates are undeserved. It's not until we add things to carbohydrates that they become high in calories. And that's the truth. It's not until you add butter and sauces to pasta that it becomes high in calories. It's not until you add butter and sour cream to potatoes that they become high in calories. Carbohydrates are good foods. They give your body its preferred form of fuel and they should always be part of a balanced meal. And that's going to separate you from fad crash diets.

MARION: That's very important. Okay. Well, Jimmy, do you think we have enough?

JIMMY: I think it's been wonderful.

PAT: Oh, I'm glad.

JIMMY: We could never have gotten all this valuable information reading textbooks. You really clarified so much. Don't you agree, honey?

MARION: Absolutely. Pat, you must be exhausted. What time is it?

JIMMY: 1:21 A.M. Do you believe it?

PAT: It's OK. This baby [patting her stomach] is a night owl. I can tell.

MARION: Pat, it must have seemed as if we were drilling you for an exam.

PAT: Well . . . I think you both knew more than you thought. There were times, however, when I felt you were testing me.

JIMMY: Maybe just a little, but you passed with flying colors. Now, you must get some sleep.

MARION: Yes, Pat, you really must. And tomorrow, I'll make you a breakfast full of protein, carbohydrates, and fat.

JIMMY: And I'll make you a chocolate cake! Only kidding, of course.

MARION: You are?

The next day, before Pat left for Durham, Marion and I kissed and hugged her. We renamed her Florence Nightingale and she loved it. We are both indebted to her. I think Marion and I slept for two days after she left. Perhaps as in all those Andy Hardy movies, we felt the crisis had passed.

I was set to do the Carson show again the following week with Joan Rivers hosting. Now, I knew I could leave without thinking about amino acids or lipids or triglycerides. Doing the show with Joan is always such a ball and I wanted to be in good form. If it hadn't been for Florence Nightingale, I might have gone on preoccupied and that is never a good idea with Joan Rivers, the quickest wit in town. I adore her and she knows it. I really think she is the funniest stand-up comic around. She and her husband Edgar and I have been friends for a long time. Going to one of their dinner parties is also a treat. The guest list is always everyone you always wanted to meet. I have never had a bad meal there or a bad time. As I said in the preface, if you want to know if Joan Rivers is as funny off camera as she is on, "read on." Well, the answer is most emphatically, yes. I also happen to think, despite her attacks on her own looks, that she is a knockout.

So, as my dear friend Joan would say, "Can we talk?" I hope this book works for you. Better yet, please let it work for you. You can do it. Remember, if I can, *you can*!

8.
Diet Menus and Recipes from the Coco Kitchen: The 21-Day Plan

Using the Diet Menus

Each day's meals are simply presented as a list of ingredients with their calorie counts. The total count for each meal is given, and then the total for each day. Following the menu plan for the day are the recipes for each meal on the menu. In some cases, the dinner menu calls for a dish that serves more than one. In this case, a note, "see preparation for full ingredients", follows beneath the dish name and calorie count and directs you to the part of the recipe that provides the number of servings and the approximate number of calories per serving, along with a full list of ingredients.

Chapter 9 provides an extensive list of foods and their calorie counts so that you can construct you own recipes or vary the ones given here. The Appendix, beginning on page 246, contains more recipes as well as suggestions for constructing your own maintenance plans, preparing and storing foods, and exercise.

First Week: Monday

	CALORIES
BREAKFAST: **SCRAMBLED EGGS**	
2 egg whites	30
½ egg yolk	35
1 teaspoon diet margarine	15
2 teaspoons skim milk powder	20
1 slice thin bread, Arnold's	40
½ teaspoon diet margarine	5
breakfast total	*145*
LUNCH: **STUFFED TOMATO WITH SPRING SALAD**	
½ cup cottage cheese	120
1 teaspoon chopped onion	0
1 teaspoon chopped carrots	0
1 teaspoon chopped green pepper	0
1 medium tomato	35
lunch total	*155*
DINNER: **SIRLOIN STEAK WITH MUSHROOMS AND WINE**	
5 ounces sirloin steak	300
½ baked potato	45
½ cup green beans	15
1 cup fresh mushrooms	20
¼ cup white wine	0
½ cup strawberries	25
dinner total	*405*
Total calories for this day	*705*

Scrambled Eggs

INGREDIENTS

  2 egg whites
  2 teaspoons skim milk powder
  ½ egg yolk*
  1 teaspoon diet margarine

PREPARATION

Combine egg whites and skim milk powder and ½ egg yolk and beat until frothy. Melt diet margarine in a nonstick frying pan. Scramble and serve.

1 slice thin sliced whole wheat Arnold bread, toasted, ½ teaspoon diet margarine for toast
Beverage: coffee or tea

* Separate egg yolk from egg white. Place yolk in glass, beat, and pour one half.

Stuffed Tomato with Spring Salad

INGREDIENTS

  ½ cup cottage cheese
  1 teaspoon chopped onion
  1 teaspoon chopped carrots
  1 teaspoon chopped green pepper
  1 medium tomato

PREPARATION

Mix the cottage cheese, onion, carrots, green pepper. Core and quarter tomato and stuff with mixture.

Broiled Sirloin Steak Dinner

PREPARATION

For 5 ounces of beef, buy 7 ounces of raw beef. Broil steak according to taste in broiler pan 3–5 inches from heat.

Cut medium-size potato in half (lengthwise). Lightly brush top with diet margarine, ¼ teaspoon or less. Place in regular or toaster oven at 375° for 35 minutes or until done.

Steam green beans for 6–10 minutes. Use lemon for flavoring and pepper to taste. If frozen, follow directions on package.

In a skillet, heat ¼ cup of wine. When hot, add mushrooms and pepper to taste. Stir for 5–8 minutes. Pour over steak.

If using frozen strawberries, use only natural—no sugar added.

First Week: Tuesday

		CALORIES
BREAKFAST:	**CEREAL**	
	1¼ cups Cheerios	110
	½ cup skim milk	45
	breakfast total	*155*
LUNCH:	**FRUIT SALAD PLATE**	
	½ cup pineapple chunks (fresh or frozen)	40
	½ tablespoon raisins	20
	¼ cup blueberries	20
	¼ cup peaches	20
	¼ cup cottage cheese	50
	lunch total	*150*
DINNER:	**SHRIMP WITH WINE AND LEMON RIND**	
	6 ounces shrimp	180
	¼ cup white wine	0
	¼ teaspoon lemon rind	0
	½ cup cooked rice	100
	4 broccoli spears	40
	½ cup carrots	20
	½ broiled grapefruit	50
	dinner total	*390*
Total calories for this day		*695*

Fruit Salad Plate

PREPARATION

Place cottage cheese in center, surround with fruit, and sprinkle with raisins.

Shrimp with Wine and Lemon Rind

INGREDIENTS

 6 ounces raw shrimp
 ½ cup cooked rice
 1 tablespoon diet margarine
 ½ cup parsley
 1 teaspoon lemon rind, minced
 ¼ cup white wine
 1 teaspoon minced garlic
 dash of black pepper

PREPARATION

Melt margarine in Teflon skillet, add wine, and bring to a simmer. Add shrimp, garlic and ¼ cup of the parsley, lemon rind and black pepper. Stir briskly for about 10 minutes. (Do not overcook). Pour over rice. Garnish with remainder of parsley.

Do not use instant rice. Cook according to directions on the box.

Broiled Half Grapefruit

PREPARATION

Place grapefruit under broiler 4 or 5 inches from heat for 5 minutes or until brown. Add a dash of nutmeg and cinnamon before serving.

First Week: Wednesday

		CALORIES
BREAKFAST:	**CEREAL**	
	½ cup oatmeal	65
	1½ tablespoons raisins	45
	½ cup skim milk	45
	breakfast total	*155*
LUNCH:	**TOMATO AND TUNA SALAD**	
	1½ ounces tuna	50
	1 tablespoon chopped egg	10
	1 tablespoon diet mayonnaise	40
	1 tablespoon chopped apple	10
	½ teaspoon chopped onion	0
	½ teaspoon dried mustard, lemon	0
	1 medium tomato	40
	lunch total	150
DINNER:	**OVEN-FRIED CHICKEN**	
	oven-fried chicken	200
	see preparation for full ingredients.	
	2 baked potato shells	50
	1 large green salad with ½ teaspoon onion, cucumber slices, and ½ tomato	45
	1 cup cauliflower	20
	1 small apple	80
	dinner total	*395*
Total calories for this day		*700*

Oatmeal

PREPARATION

Cook oatmeal according to directions on box. Do not use instant oatmeal. Use rolled oats.

Tomato and Tuna Salad

INGREDIENTS

1½ ounces tuna
1 tablespoon chopped egg
1 tablespoon diet mayonnaise
1 tablespoon chopped apple
½ tablespoon chopped onion
1 tablespoon chopped celery
½ teaspoon dry mustard, lemon
1 medium tomato, quartered

PREPARATION

Mix all ingredients.

Oven-Fried Chicken

INGREDIENTS

12 ounces raw chicken breast, split and skinned
1 slice thin bread, Arnold's
(toasted and made into bread crumbs)
¼ cup dehydrated onions
1 teaspoon parmesan cheese
2 egg whites
dash of black pepper

PREPARATION

Mix bread crumbs, onions, parmesan cheese and black pepper. Dip chicken in egg white, then coat with breading. In a shallow pan, lined with foil, place chicken breast side up and bake in 375° oven for 40 minutes or until golden brown.

Cut one medium baked potato lengthwise and scoop out inside with a spoon, leaving a thin layer of flesh. Rub inside lightly with diet margarine (¼ teaspoon or less) and bake in oven or toaster oven at 375° for 30 minutes or until golden brown. Serves 2. Approximate number of calories per serving: 200.

First Week: Thursday

		CALORIES
BREAKFAST:	**CEREAL**	
	¾ cup Special K	70
	½ cup skim milk	45
	½ cup blueberries	45
	breakfast total	*160*
LUNCH:	**EGG SALAD PLATE**	
	1 hard boiled egg, chopped	75
	1 tablespoon diet mayonnaise	40
	½ tablespoon chopped onion	10
	1 tablespoon chopped celery	0
	½ teaspoon dry mustard	0
	½ medium tomato diced	20
	lunch total	*145*
DINNER:	**SWEDISH MEATBALLS WITH WINE SAUCE**	
	Swedish meatballs see full ingredients on preparation page.	300
	4 broccoli spears with lemon	40
	½ baked acorn squash	45
	1 teaspoon diet margarine	10
	½ teaspoon cinnamon	0
	dinner total	*395*
Total calories for this day		*700*

Egg Salad Plate

INGREDIENTS

1 hard boiled egg, chopped
1 tablespoon diet mayonnaise
½ tablespoon chopped onion
1 tablespoon chopped celery
½ teaspoon dry mustard
½ medium tomato diced

PREPARATION

Mix ingredients and serve on a lettuce leaf.

Swedish Meatballs

INGREDIENTS

8 ounces raw lean chopped veal
½ teaspoon dry dill
½ cup onion
½ slice thinly sliced bread
1 ounce skim milk
¼ teaspoon nutmeg
1 egg (beaten)

Sauce

6 ounces skim milk
1 tablespoon flour
1 teaspoon diet margarine
2 ounces white wine

PREPARATION

Soak bread in skim milk. Add veal, onion, egg, dill, nutmeg. Prepare into two-ounce balls: 3 meatballs per serving. Bake at 350° for ½ hour or until done.

Make sauce while meat is baking:

Melt margarine. Add to flour. Add a little cold milk. Mix well. Heat the rest of the milk. Add in margarine, flour, cold milk mixture. Stir vigorously. Add wine, margarine. After simmering, should be 5–6 ounces of sauce. Two ounces is approximately 35 calories. Serving size: 3 (2 oz.) meatballs with ¼ cup sauce. Serves 2. Approximate calories: 300 per serving.

First Week: Friday

		CALORIES
BREAKFAST:	**CEREAL**	
	¾ cup puffed wheat	30
	½ cup skim milk	45
	1 small orange	80
	breakfast total	*155*
LUNCH:	**PITA SANDWICH STUFFED WITH TURKEY**	
	½ slice small pita bread	40
	1 ounce cooked turkey, diced	50
	¼ cup alfalfa sprouts	5
	1 slice tomato	5
	5 slices cucumber	5
	2 ounces low-calorie dressing	0
	½ banana	45
	lunch total	*150*
DINNER:	**FLOUNDER WITH CORNFLAKE CRUMBS**	
	9 ounces flounder	180
	1 tablespoon diet mayonnaise	40
	2 tablespoons crushed cornflakes	40
	½ cup rice	100
	salad with tomato and onion and green pepper	40
	dinner total	*400*
Total calories for this day		705

Pita Sandwich

INGREDIENTS

$\frac{1}{2}$ slice small pita bread
1 ounce cooked turkey, diced
$\frac{1}{4}$ cup alfalfa sprouts
1 slice tomato
5 slices cucumber
2 ounces low-calorie dressing

PREPARATION

Place ingredients inside pocket bread and top with dressing.

Flounder With Cornflake Crumbs

INGREDIENTS

9 ounces flounder
1 tablespoon diet mayonnaise
2 tablespoons crushed cornflakes

PREPARATION

Place flounder in spray-coated baking dish. Spread diet mayonnaise on the top of the fish. Sprinkle with cornflake crumbs. Bake in preheated 450° oven for about 10 minutes or until fish flakes when tested with a fork.

First Week: Saturday

	CALORIES
BREAKFAST: **CEREAL**	
1 banana	90
1 serving puffed wheat or puffed rice	30
with ½ cup skim milk	<u>45</u>
breakfast total	*165*
LUNCH: **SPINACH SOUFFLE**	
½ cup cooked spinach	25
1 teaspoon parmesan cheese	25
1 teaspoon diet margarine	10
3 egg whites	45
½ cup strawberries	<u>25</u>
lunch total	*130*
DINNER: **CHICKEN ROSEMARY**	
chicken rosemary see full ingredients on preparation page	300
½ cup mashed potatoes	45
½ cup spinach	20
¼ cantaloupe	<u>30</u>
dinner total	*405*
Total calories for this day	*700*

Spinach Souffle

INGREDIENTS

- ½ cup cooked spinach
- 3 egg whites, whipped
- 1 teaspoon dehydrated onion
- 1 teaspoon parmesan cheese
- ½ teaspoon diet margarine

PREPARATION

Cook spinach until tender. Drain. Add chopped onion and spinach and fold in the egg white. Bake in a 350° oven for approximately 35 minutes. Use ½ teaspoon margarine to coat 5 × 5 inch casserole oven-proof dish.

Chicken Rosemary

INGREDIENTS

- 12 ounces raw chicken breast, skin removed
- ¼ teaspoon finely crushed rosemary
- ¼ teaspoon garlic powder
- ½ teaspoon paprika
- ½ teaspoon dehydrated onion flakes
- ½ tablespoon lemon juice
- 2 tablespoons vinegar
- ½ cup sliced fresh mushrooms

PREPARATION

Combine first four ingredients. Separately combine next three ingredients. Place chicken bone side up in a baking dish. Sprinkle with half of the herb mixture. Turn chicken over and sprinkle with the rest of the herb mixture. Spoon vinegar and lemon juice over chicken. Cover and refrigerate

at least 4 hours before cooking, basting occasionally. Bake
covered at 350° for 30 minutes. Top the chicken with
sliced mushrooms and baste thoroughly with pan juices.
Cover again and bake 15 minutes. Remove cover and cook
10–15 minutes longer if you desire a browned top. Serves 2.
Approximate number of calories per serving: 310.

Mashed Potatoes

Wash and peel potato. Cut in half and place in boiling water
until cooked, about 15 minutes. Remove, drain, and mash
with 1 tablespoon skim milk, ½ teaspoon diet margarine,
and a dash of pepper.

First Week: Sunday

		CALORIES
BREAKFAST:	**CEREAL**	
	4 ounces orange juice	55
	1 serving puffed wheat or puffed rice	30
	4 ounces skim milk	45
	¼ cup blueberries	20
	breakfast total	*150*
LUNCH:	**ZUCCHINI SOUFFLE**	
	½ cup cooked zucchini	25
	1 teaspoon parmesan cheese	25
	1 teaspoon diet margarine	10
	3 egg whites	45
	½ cup strawberries	25
	lunch total	*130*
DINNER:	**VEAL LOAF**	
	veal loaf	325
	see full ingredients	
	on preparation page.	
	Red and green bell peppers	40
	roasted potatoes	40
	dinner total	*405*
Total calories for this day		*685*

Zucchini Souffle

INGREDIENTS

1 cup cooked zucchini, diced
3 egg whites whipped
1 teaspoon dehydrated onion
1 teaspoon parmesan cheese
½ tablespoon diet margarine

PREPARATION

Cook zucchini until tender. Drain. Add chopped onion and zucchini and fold in the egg white. Bake in a 350° oven for approximately 35 minutes.

Veal Loaf

INGREDIENTS

2 pounds ground veal
1 cup chopped fresh mushrooms
1½ cups fresh bread crumbs
½ cup imitation sour cream
1 small onion, minced
1½ cups shredded carrots
2 egg whites
1 teaspoon bottled steak sauce
¼ tablespoon fresh or 1 teaspoon dried dill
½ teaspoon black pepper, or to taste

PREPARATION

Preheat oven to 350°. Place all the ingredients in a large bowl and mix well. Pour into 9″ × 5″ loaf pan and bake for 1¼ hours. Remove from oven and let stand at room temperature for 5 minutes. Pour off liquid and reserve. Loosen loaf from pan and invert onto warm platter. Serve with reserved liquid. Serves 6. Approximate calories per serving: 325.

Roasted Peppers and Potatoes

INGREDIENTS

  6 green bell peppers
  6 red bell peppers
  2 medium-size potatoes
  1 tablespoon soy sauce
  ½ cup water
  1 tablespoon polyunsaturated oil
  2 tablespoons onion flakes

PREPARATION

Preheat oven to 350°. Wash and core peppers and cut into thin strips. Peel and parboil potatoes; cut in half and then lengthwise into strips. Place peppers and potatoes in roasting pan. Sprinkle with soy sauce, water, oil, and onion flakes. Mix well. Bake for 1¼ hours (can be cooked at the same time as the veal loaf), turning pieces occasionally. Arrange on platter around veal loaf.

Second Week: Monday

		CALORIES
BREAKFAST:	**SCRAMBLED EGGS**	
	2 egg whites	30
	½ egg yolk	35
	1 teaspoon diet margarine	15
	1 teaspoon skim milk powder	20
	1 slice thin bread, Arnold's	40
	½ teaspoon diet margarine for toast	5
	breakfast total	*145*
LUNCH:	**FRUIT SALAD PLATE**	
	¼ cantaloupe	30
	½ banana	40
	½ cup strawberries	25
	1 tablespoon raisins	30
	4 tablespoons low-fat yogurt	40
	lunch total	*165*
DINNER:	**SIRLOIN STEAK DINNER WITH MUSHROOMS**	
	5 ounces sirloin	300
	½ baked potato	45
	½ cup green beans	15
	1 cup fresh mushrooms	20
	¼ cup white wine	0
	dinner total	*380*
Total calories for this day		*690*

Scrambled Eggs

INGREDIENTS

> 2 *egg whites*
> 1 *teaspoon skim milk powder*
> ½ *egg yolk**
> 1 *teaspoon diet margarine*

PREPARATION

Combine skim milk powder and egg whites and ½ egg yolk and beat until frothy. Melt diet margarine in a nonstick frying pan. Scramble and serve.

*Separate egg yolk from egg white. Place yolk in glass, beat, and pour out half.

Fruit Salad Plate

PREPARATION

Slice fruit. Serve on plate. Add yogurt and sprinkle raisins on top.

Broiled Sirlon Steak Dinner with Mushrooms

PREPARATION

For 5 ounces of beef, buy 7 ounces of raw beef. Broil steak according to taste in broiler pan 3–5 inches from heat.

Cut medium-size potato in half (lengthwise). Lightly brush top with diet margarine, ¼ teaspoon or less. Place in regular or toaster oven at 375° for 35 minutes or until done.

Steam green beans for 6–10 minutes. Use lemon for flavoring and pepper to taste. If frozen, follow directions on package.

In a skillet, heat ¼ cup of wine. When hot, add mushrooms and pepper to taste. Stir for 5–8 minutes. Pour over steak.

Second Week: Tuesday

		CALORIES
BREAKFAST:	**CEREAL**	
	½ cup oatmeal	65
	½ cup skim milk	45
	1½ tablespoons raisins	<u>45</u>
	breakfast total	*155*
LUNCH:	**EGG SALAD PLATE**	
	1 hard boiled egg, chopped	75
	1 tablespoon diet mayonnaise	40
	½ tablespoon chopped onion	0
	1 tablespoon chopped celery	0
	½ teaspoon dry mustard	0
	½ medium tomato, diced	<u>20</u>
	lunch total	*135*
DINNER:	**CHICKEN DIJON**	
	chicken breast	300
	¼ cup rice	50
	6 fresh asparagus with lemon sauce	25
	½ cup strawberries	<u>25</u>
	dinner total	*400*
Total calories for this day		*690*

Egg Salad Plate

INGREDIENTS

1   hard boiled egg, chopped
1   tablespoon diet mayonnaise
½   tablespoon chopped onion
1   tablespoon chopped celery
½   teaspoon dry mustard
½   medium tomato, diced

PREPARATION

Mix ingredients and serve on lettuce leaf.

Chicken Dijon

INGREDIENTS

Chicken breast
1   tablespoon diet margarine
Dijon sauce

PREPARATION

Brown chicken on both sides in 1 tablespoon margarine in a
Teflon skillet. Place chicken breast side down and pour
Dijon sauce over chicken. Cover and cook for 45 minutes.
   Dijon sauce: Mix in a bowl:

2   tablespoons mustard
1   cup water
1   clove garlic, minced
juice of 1 lemon

Second Week: Wednesday

		CALORIES
BREAKFAST:	**CEREAL**	
	¾ cup puffed rice	30
	½ cup skim milk	45
	1 small banana	80
	breakfast total	155
LUNCH:	**FRUIT DELUXE**	
	½ cantaloupe	60
	1 cup strawberries	50
	¼ cup cottage cheese	60
	lunch total	170
DINNER:	**VEAL PARMESAN**	
	4 ounces veal (2–3 slices), pounded thin	240
	1 teaspoon parmesan cheese	30
	2 teaspoons diet margarine	20
	½ teaspoon garlic, minced	0
	noodles with poppy seed	50
	tomato and mozzarella	30
	dinner total	370
Total calories for this day		695

Fruit Deluxe

PREPARATION

Fill ½ cantaloupe with cottage cheese and berries and serve.

Veal Parmesan

INGREDIENTS

    4 ounces veal
    1 teaspoon parmesan cheese
    2 teaspoons diet margarine
    ½ teaspoon garlic, minced

PREPARATION

Season veal with black pepper and garlic. Rub cheese on both sides of cutlets. Melt margarine in a Teflon frying pan and, when hot, saute veal on both sides, about 5 minutes.

Serve with ½ cup of egg noodles. Mix with 1 teaspoon diet margarine and 1 teaspoon poppy seed.

On a bed of lettuce place 3 slices of tomato with low-cal dressing and 1 slice of part-skim milk mozzarella cheese. Sprinkle with fresh basil.

Second Week: Thursday

		CALORIES
BREAKFAST:	**CEREAL**	
	¾ cup Product 19	110
	½ cup skim milk	45
	breakfast total	*155*
LUNCH:	**LARGE MIXED SALAD**	
	6 ounces lettuce, with cucumber, tomato, onion, and raw zucchini	50
	½ grapefruit	50
	lunch total	*150*
DINNER:	**MEAT LOAF DINNER**	
	meat loaf	300
	see preparation page for full ingredients.	
	8 ounces lean ground round	
	2 baked potato shells	50
	4 broccoli spears	40
	dinner total	*390*
Total calories for this day		*695*

Large Mixed Salad

PREPARATION

Shred the lettuce, add sliced vegetables. Use 2 tablespoons low-cal dressing. Mix and serve.

Meat Loaf

INGREDIENTS

8 ounces lean, raw beef, ground round
1 slice bread in small cubes
1 egg
¼ cup green pepper
¼ cup onion
½ tomato, diced

PREPARATION

Mix all ingredients. Place in small, 1-quart casserole dish. Bake at 375° for 1 hour. Serves 2. Approximate calories per serving: 300.

Second Week: Friday

		CALORIES
BREAKFAST:	**SCRAMBLED EGGS**	
	2 egg whites	30
	½ egg yolk	35
	1 teaspoon diet margarine	15
	1 slice thin bread, Arnold's	40
	½ teaspoon diet margarine	5
	breakfast total	*125*
LUNCH:	**PITA SANDWICH STUFFED WITH TURKEY**	
	½ slice small pita bread	40
	1 ounce cooked turkey, diced	50
	¼ cup alfalfa sprouts	5
	1 slice tomato	5
	5 slices cucumber	5
	2 ounces low-calorie dressing	0
	½ banana	45
	lunch total	*150*
DINNER:	**TUNA-COTTAGE CHEESE CASSEROLE**	
	3 ounces tuna fish, drained	90
	¼ cup cottage cheese	60
	2 egg whites	30
	1 tablespoon each, onion and green pepper, chopped	10
	Spices: celery seed, dry mustard	0
	Large salad with special dressing	50
	½ cup rice	100
	Strawberry and blueberry special with yogurt topping	55
	dinner total	*395*
Total calories for this day		*670*

Scrambled Eggs

INGREDIENTS

  2 egg whites
  2 teaspoons skim milk powder
  ½ egg yolk*
  1 teaspoon diet margarine

PREPARATION

Combine skim milk powder and egg whites and ½ egg yolk
and beat until frothy. Melt diet margarine in a nonstick
frying pan. Scramble and serve.

1 slice thin whole wheat Arnold's bread, toasted
½ teaspoon diet margarine for toast
Beverage: coffee or tea

*Separate egg yolk from egg white. Place yolk in glass, beat, and pour out
half.

Pita Sandwich Stuffed with Turkey

INGREDIENTS

  ½ slice small pita bread
  1 ounce cooked turkey, diced
  ¼ cup alfalfa sprouts
  1 slice tomato
  5 slices cucumber
  2 ounces low-calorie dressing

PREPARATION

Place ingredients inside pocket bread and top with dressing.

Tuna-Cottage Cheese Casserole

INGREDIENTS

3 ounces tuna fish, drained
¼ cup cottage cheese
2 egg whites
1 tablespoon each, onion and green pepper, chopped
Spices: celery seed, dry mustard

PREPARATION

Combine tuna, cottage cheese, onion, and any spices you
desire. Beat egg whites until stiff. Fold mixture into beaten
egg whites. Pour mixture into a baking dish. Sprinkle with
paprika. Bake ½ hour at 350°. Broil to brown after baking.
Garnish with lemon wedges and parsley.

Second Week: Saturday

	CALORIES
BREAKFAST: **MUSHROOM OMELET**	
3 egg whites	45
1 teaspoon diet margarine	10
1 cup mushrooms	20
1 slice thin bread, Arnold's	40
½ teaspoon diet margarine	5
breakfast total	*120*
LUNCH: **HOT VEGETABLE PLATE**	
½ cup broccoli	20
½ cup summer squash	15
½ cup beets	30
¼ cup cottage cheese	50
fruit and yogurt	30
lunch total	*145*
DINNER: **BEEF STEW**	
beef stew	340
see full ingredients on preparation page.	
½ baked squash and large salad	80
dinner total	*420*
Total calories for this day	*685*

Mushroom Omelet

INGREDIENTS

> 3 egg whites
> 1 teaspoon diet margarine
> 1 cup cooked mushrooms

PREPARATION

Beat egg whites. Melt margarine in a nonstick frying pan.
Pour in egg mixture. Have heat on medium. Let egg whites
sit and cook. As egg whites become less and less clear, the
edges will brown and air bubbles will come through. Add
mushrooms. As the edges brown, place a spatula underneath and begin to separate egg white from bottom of frying
pan. Do not turn over until the egg whites are brown all the
way around and air bubbles are coming through the whole
egg white. When you see the air bubbles come all the way
through the egg white, flip, either in half or like a pancake.
  Toast bread and use ½ teaspoon margarine on it.

Hot Vegetable Plate

PREPARATION

Steam vegetables, center cottage cheese on plate, and surround with vegetables.

Fruit and Yogurt

Mix ¼ cup strawberries with three tablespoons yogurt. Stir.
Chill and serve.

Beef Stew

INGREDIENTS

1 pound lean beef
2 tablespoons flour
1 tablespoon oil
1 pound stewing tomatoes
1 bay leaf
1 medium onion, chopped
2 medium potatoes, diced
1 cup carrots, chopped
1 stalk celery, diced
Worcestershire sauce
Beef bouillon cube

PREPARATION

Cut beef into 1½ inch cubes. Shake in plastic bag with flour.
Carefully brown in oil, preferably in Teflon pan over medium
heat. Transfer to stewing pot and add tomatoes, Worcestershire sauce, onion, celery, bay leaf, pepper, and 1½ cups
water. Simmer, covered, 1½ hours. Then add beef bouillon
cube, potatoes, and carrots. Add ½ to 1 cup water, depending on thickness of stew, and continue to simmer, covered,
for ½ hour. Remove cover, cook down to desired thickness.
Divide into four equal portions and serve. Serves 4. Approximate calories per serving: 340.

Baked Squash

INGREDIENTS

1 acorn squash
dash cinnamon
1 teaspoon diet margarine

PREPARATION

Cut squash in half, remove seeds. Place squash cut side down. Bake at 350° for 40 minutes. Brush with margarine, sprinkle with cinnamon. (Serves 2.)

Salad

Toss ¼ wedge lettuce, ½ tomato, sliced, and a dash of pepper. Add 2 tablespoons of low-cal dressing.

Second Week: Sunday

		CALORIES
BREAKFAST:	**COTTAGE CHEESE OMELET**	

¼ cup cottage cheese · 50
3 egg whites · 45
1 teaspoon diet margarine · 10
1 slice thin bread, Arnold's (toasted) · 40
½ teaspoon diet margarine · 5

breakfast total · *150*

LUNCH: **SHRIMP COCKTAIL**

4 ounces cooked shrimp (cooled) · 120
1 ounce cocktail sauce · 5
½ tomato · 20
Vegetable strips as follows: 3 celery, 3 green pepper, 3 carrot, 3 zucchini · 15

lunch total · *160*

DINNER: **CHICKEN WITH WINE SAUCE, APPLES, AND RAISINS**

12 ounces chicken breast · 300
½ cup mashed potatoes · 40
½ cup spinach · 30
½ cup strawberries with 1 tablespoon of yogurt topping · 30

dinner total · *400*

Total calories for this day · *710*

Cottage Cheese Omelet

INGREDIENTS

> 3 egg whites
> 1 teaspoon diet margarine
> ¼ cup cottage cheese
> 1 slice thinly sliced bread, toasted

PREPARATION

Beat egg whites. Melt margarine in a nonstick frying pan. Pour in egg mixture. Have heat on medium. Let egg whites sit and cook. As egg whites become less and less clear, the edges will brown and air bubbles will come through. Add cottage cheese. As the edges brown, place a spatula underneath and begin to separate egg white from bottom of frying pan. Yet do not turn over until the egg whites are brown all the way around and air bubbles are coming through the whole egg white. When you see the air bubbles come all the way through the egg white, flip, either in half or like a pancake.

Shrimp Cocktail

PREPARATION

Place raw shrimp, shelled and cleaned, in boiling water for about 5 minutes. Drain and cool. Place on platter and surround with vegetable strips and tomato.

To make cocktail sauce, mix ¼ cup tomato (peeled and mashed), ¼ teaspoon crushed red pepper, and ¼ teaspoon horseradish. Chill.

Chicken with Wine Sauce, Apples, and Raisins

INGREDIENTS

> 12 ounces raw chicken with bone and fat, remove skin
> 1/4 cup chopped apple
> 1/2 tablespoon raisins
> 1/4 cup white wine

PREPARATION

Skin chicken. Place in closed casserole dish. Sprinkle chopped apple and raisins on top of chicken. Pour wine over all. Bake at 350° for 30 minutes or until done. While baking, ladle sauce back on top of chicken.

Third Week: Monday

		CALORIES
BREAKFAST:	**CEREAL**	
	½ cup oatmeal	65
	1½ tablespoons raisins	45
	½ cup skim milk	45
	breakfast total	*155*
LUNCH:	**RAW VEGETABLE PLATTER**	
	½ cup broccoli	20
	1 cup zucchini	30
	½ cup cauliflower	20
	¼ cup cottage cheese	50
	½ cup fresh strawberries	25
	lunch total	*145*
DINNER:	**SIRLOIN STEAK DINNER**	
	5 ounces sirloin steak	300
	½ baked potato	45
	½ cup green beans	15
	1 cup fresh mushrooms	20
	¼ cup white wine	0
	½ cup fresh strawberries	25
	dinner total	*405*
Total calories for this day		*705*

Raw Vegetable Platter

PREPARATION

Wash vegetables and use the broccoli flowers. Do the same with the cauliflower. Wash but do not peel zucchini. Slice off one end of zucchini, then slice enough for ½ cup. Arrange on plate. Center cottage cheese.

Broiled Sirloin Steak Dinner

PREPARATION

For 5 ounces of beef, buy 7 ounces of raw beef. Broil steak according to taste in broiler pan 3–5 inches from heat.

Cut medium-size potato in half (lengthwise). Lightly brush top with diet margarine, ¼ teaspoon or less. Place in regular or toaster oven at 375° for 35 minutes or until done.

Steam green beans for 6–10 minutes. Use lemon for flavoring and pepper to taste. If frozen, follow directions on package.

In a skillet, heat ¼ cup of wine. When hot, add mushrooms and pepper to taste. Stir for 5–8 minutes. Pour over steak.

If using frozen strawberries, use only natural—no sugar added.

Third Week: Tuesday

		CALORIES
BREAKFAST:	**SCRAMBLED EGGS**	
	2 egg whites	30
	½ egg yolk	35
	1 teaspoon diet margarine	15
	2 teaspoons skim milk powder	20
	1 slice thin bread, Arnold's	40
	½ teaspoon diet margarine for toast	5
	Beverage	
	breakfast total	*145*
LUNCH:	**SPRING SALAD**	
	½ cup cottage cheese	120
	1 teaspoon chopped onion	0
	1 teaspoon chopped carrots	0
	1 teaspoon chopped green pepper	0
	1 medium tomato	35
	lunch total	*155*
DINNER:	**BROILED CHICKEN WITH LEMON AND CINNAMON**	
	12 ounces chicken breast, split and skinned	300
	1 cup sauteed mushrooms	35
	1 cup green beans	25
	½ baked potato	50
	dinner total	*410*
Total calories for this day		*710*

Scrambled Eggs

INGREDIENTS

> 2 egg whites
> 2 teaspoons skim milk powder
> ½ egg yolk
> 1 teaspoon diet margarine

PREPARATION

Combine skim milk powder and egg whites and ½ egg yolk and beat until frothy. Melt diet margarine in a nonstick frying pan. Scramble and serve.

1 slice thin sliced whole wheat Arnold bread, toasted
½ teaspoon diet margarine for toast
Beverage: coffee or tea

Stuffed Tomato with Spring Salad

INGREDIENTS

> ½ cup cottage cheese
> 1 teaspoon chopped onion
> 1 teaspoon chopped carrots
> 1 teaspoon chopped green pepper
> 1 medium tomato

PREPARATION

Mix the cottage cheese, onion, carrots, green pepper. Core and quarter tomato and stuff with mixture.

Chicken with Lemon and Cinnamon

INGREDIENTS

- *12 ounces chicken, one whole breast, split, skinned and with bone*
- *2 lemons, squeezed*
- *1 tablespoon oil*
- *1 clove garlic, minced*
- *1 teaspoon oregano*
- *2 tablespoons ground cinnamon*

PREPARATION

In a mixing bowl add: the lemons, oil, garlic, oregano, and cinnamon. Mix well. After chicken is broiled, place on a platter and pour mixture over chicken.

Third Week: Wednesday

		CALORIES
BREAKFAST:	**CEREAL**	
	¾ cup cream of wheat*	65
	½ cup skim milk	45
	½ medium orange	40
	breakfast total	*150*
LUNCH:	**EGG SALAD PLATE**	
	1 hard boiled egg, chopped	75
	1 tablespoon diet mayonnaise	40
	½ tablespoon chopped onion	0
	1 tablespoon chopped celery	0
	½ teaspoon dry mustard	0
	½ medium tomato, diced	20
	lunch total	*145*
DINNER:	**FISH CREOLE**	
	Fish creole	200
	½ cup rice (cooked)	100
	1 cup spinach (steamed or frozen)	40
	½ cantaloupe	60
	dinner total	*400*

Total calories for this day   *695*

*Cook according to package directions.

Egg Salad Plate

INGREDIENTS

1 hard boiled egg, chopped
1 tablespoon diet mayonnaise
½ tablespoon chopped onion
1 tablespoon chopped celery
½ teaspoon dry mustard
½ medium tomato, diced

PREPARATION

Mix all ingredients. Chill and serve.

Fish Creole

INGREDIENTS

8 ounces raw (5 ounces cooked) low-fat fish
½ tomato, blended
2 tablespoons chopped green pepper
2 tablespoons choppped onion
2 tablespoons chopped celery
Lemon juice, paprika, oregano, sweet basil

PREPARATION

Place fish in pan. Pour lemon juice over it, and sprinkle green pepper, onion, and celery. Pour on blended tomato. Add paprika, oregano, sweet basil. Bake at 350° for ½ hour. Serve hot.

Third Week: Thursday

	CALORIES
BREAKFAST: **CEREAL**	
¾ cup Cheerios	110
½ cup skim milk	45
breakfast total	*155*
LUNCH: **TUNA FISH SALAD PLATE**	
1½ ounces tuna	50
1 tablespoon chopped egg	10
1 tablespoon diet mayonnaise	40
1 tablespoon chopped apple	10
½ tablespoon chopped onion	0
1 tablespoon chopped celery	0
1 teaspoon dry mustard	0
1 medium tomato, quartered	40
lunch total	*150*
DINNER: **STUFFED PEPPER**	
½ cup cooked rice	100
2½ ounces beef	150
2 tablespoons tomato sauce	10
1 small green pepper	10
1 cup chopped broccoli	40
4 asparagus spears	20
2 tablespoons vinaigrette	10
½ grapefruit	50
dinner total	*390*
Total calories for this day	695

Tuna Fish Salad Plate

INGREDIENTS

1½ ounces tuna
1 tablespoon chopped egg
1 tablespoon diet mayonnaise
1 tablespoon chopped apple
½ tablespoon chopped onion
1 tablespoon chopped celery
1 teaspoon dry mustard
1 medium tomato, quartered

PREPARATION

Mix all ingredients. Chill and serve.

Stuffed Pepper

INGREDIENTS

½ cup cooked rice
2½ ounces cooked beef
2 tablespoons tomato sauce
1 small green pepper

PREPARATION

Mix rice, cooked meat, sauce, and any additional spices. Spoon mixture into green pepper which has been cored and blanched. Bake for 30 minutes at 350° or until done. For variety, place stuffed pepper in saucepan and simmer in 4 ounces of tomato sauce. Add additional tomato sauce after baking for flavor.

Third Week: Friday

		CALORIES
BREAKFAST:	**CEREAL**	
	¾ cup puffed wheat	30
	½ cup skim milk	45
	1 small orange	80
	breakfast total	*155*
LUNCH:	**PITA SANDWICH STUFFED WITH TURKEY**	
	½ slice small pita bread	40
	1 ounce cooked turkey, diced	50
	¼ cup alfalfa sprouts	5
	1 slice tomato	5
	5 slices cucumber	5
	2 ounces low-calorie dressing	0
	½ banana	45
	lunch total	*150*
DINNER:	**LOBSTER DINNER**	
	1 10-ounce lobster	150
	1 teaspoon margarine	35
	2 potato shells	50
	1 tablespoon melted diet margarine	50
	large salad	25
	dinner total	*310*
Total calories for this day		*615*

Pita Sandwich Stuffed with Turkey

INGREDIENTS

> ½ small pita bread
> 1 ounce cooked turkey, diced
> ¼ cup alfalfa sprouts
> 1 slice tomato
> 5 slices cucumber
> 2 ounces low-calorie dressing

PREPARATION

Place ingredients inside pocket bread and top with dressing.

Lobster

INGREDIENTS

> 1 10-ounce lobster (yields 4–5 ounces cooked meat)
> 1 teaspoon margarine

PREPARATION

Cut shell with poultry shears (or a sharp scissors). Break off last two pieces of shell near tail. Turn. Push down gently to crack spine. Turn. Gently pry lobster meat away from shell. (Do not crack shell.) Pull lobster meat out of shell. Support with palm of your hand. Rinse. Make three partial cuts down meat to widen. Spread. (This is called fantailing.) Replace meat on top of shell. Fan out the tail of the shell. (This makes it look pretty.) Season with one pat margarine, pinch of lemon, and paprika. Bake at 450° for 15–20 minutes.

Third Week: Saturday

		CALORIES
BREAKFAST:	**MUSHROOM OMELET**	
	3 egg whites	45
	1 teaspoon diet margarine	10
	1 cup mushrooms	20
	1 slice thin bread, Arnold's	40
	breakfast total	*115*
LUNCH:	**HOT VEGETABLE PLATE**	
	½ cup broccoli	20
	½ cup summer squash	15
	½ cup beets	30
	¼ cup cottage cheese	50
	fruit and yogurt	30
	lunch total	*145*
DINNER:	**OVEN-FRIED CHICKEN & BAKED SQUASH**	
	oven-fried chicken	200
	see preparation for full ingredients	
	½ baked squash	50
	large salad with tomato, onions, and lettuce	50
	½ cup green beans	20
	½ cantaloupe	60
	dinner total	*380*
Total calories for this day		*640*

Mushroom Omelet

INGREDIENTS

> 3 egg whites
> 1 teaspoon diet margarine
> 1 cup cooked mushrooms

Beat egg whites. Melt margarine in a nonstick frying pan.
Pour in egg mixture. Have heat on medium. Let egg whites
sit and cook. As egg whites become less and less clear, the
edges will brown and air bubbles will come through. Add
mushrooms. As the edges brown, place a spatula underneath and begin to separate egg white from bottom of frying
pan. Yet do not turn over until the egg whites are brown all
the way around and air bubbles are coming through the
whole egg white. When you see the air bubbles come all the
way through the egg white, flip, either in half or like a
pancake.

Toast bread and use ½ teaspoon of margarine.

Hot Vegetable Plate

PREPARATION

Steam vegetables, center cottage cheese on plate, and surround with vegetables.

Fruit and Yogurt

Mix ¼ cup strawberries with 3 tablespoons yogurt. Stir,
chill, and serve.

Oven-Fried Chicken

INGREDIENTS

  12 ounces raw chicken breast, split (bone in) and skinned
  1 slice thin bread, Arnold's (toasted and made into bread
    crumbs)
  1/4 cup dehydrated onion
  1 teaspoon parmesan cheese
  2 egg whites
  dash of black pepper

PREPARATION

Mix bread crumbs, onions, parmesan cheese, and black pepper. Dip chicken in egg white, then coat with breading. In a shallow pan lined with foil, place chicken breast side up and bake in 375° oven for 40 minutes or until golden brown. Serves 2. Approximate number of calories per serving: 200.

Baked Squash

INGREDIENTS

  1 acorn squash
  dash cinnamon
  1 teaspoon diet margarine

PREPARATION

Cut squash in half, remove seeds. Place squash in pan, cut side down. Bake at 350° for 40 minutes. Brush with margarine, sprinkle with cinnamon.

Third Week: Sunday

		CALORIES
BREAKFAST:	**CEREAL**	
	¾ cup puffed rice	30
	½ cup skim milk	45
	2 tablespoons raisins	<u>50</u>
	breakfast total	*125*
LUNCH:	**ASPARAGUS SOUFFLE**	
	½ cup cooked asparagus	25
	1 teaspoon parmesan cheese	25
	1 teaspoon diet margarine	10
	3 egg whites	45
	½ banana	<u>45</u>
	lunch total	*150*
DINNER:	**STUFFED EGGPLANT**	
	Eggplant stuffed with veal and beef	380
	see preparation for full ingredients.	
	½ cup steamed carrots	20
	½ cup cooked spinach	20
	½ cup strawberries	<u>25</u>
	dinner total	*445*
Total calories for this day		*720*

Asparagus Souffle

INGREDIENTS

1 cup cooked asparagus, cooled and mashed
3 egg whites, whipped
1 teaspoon dehydrated onion
1 teaspoon parmesan cheese
1/2 teaspoon diet margarine

PREPARATION

Steam asparagus till tender, cool and mash. Add chopped onion to asparagus and fold in egg white. Sprinkle parmesan cheese on top. Use margarine to coat a 5 × 5 inch oven proof casserole dish. Bake in a 350° oven for approximately 35 minutes.

Stuffed Eggplant

INGREDIENTS

1 large eggplant
1 cup chopped mushrooms
1 cup chopped onions
4 ounces chopped lean beef
4 ounces chopped lean veal
1/4 cup bread crumbs
1 teaspoon basil
1/2 teaspoon chervil
2 tablespoons of diet margarine
2 beaten egg whites
1/4 cup cooked tomatoes
1/2 teaspoon pepper
2 tablespoons chopped parsley
1 teaspoon parmesan cheese

PREPARATION

Preheat oven to 350°. Wash eggplant and cut in half lengthwise. Remove the pulp, leaving about ½ inch of the outer shell. Saute mushrooms, onions, meat, and seasonings in diet margarine, adding the eggplant pulp which has been diced. Cook until the meat is slightly done. Transfer to mixing bowl and add bread crumbs, cheese, egg whites, and tomatoes. Mix well as you would with a meat loaf. Spoon mixture into the eggplant shells and place in a lightly oiled ovenproof dish. Bake 35 minutes. Garnish with parsley. This makes a really different and delicious main course. Serves 2. Approximate calories: 380 per serving.

9. Calorie-Counter: The Star of the Show

Calories

You have discovered by now that calories are the star of this show. In a sense it's natural casting. If you are going to lose weight, you have to count calories and then cut them. If you are going to maintain the weight loss, you are going to have to know how many calories there are in the servings of food you want to structure into your menu. And when you cook for yourself and for your guests using the recipes in this book, you are going to be calorie-conscious—you're going to *have* to be!

Well, here it is! What follows is the most complete listing of calorie values you are going to find anywhere: foods of all sorts and descriptions, with serving size and calories. When you want to check back to find the number of calories in such Italian wonders as ricotta, mozzarella, or provolone for one of the recipes, they'll be there. Or if you want to structure in a glass of champagne, you'll find it (as a dinner wine). Even a piece of pizza.

This formidable table of calorie content contains the values given in the U.S. Department of Agriculture's bulletin *Nutritive Value of Foods*. What could be more authoritative or dependable?

So, start counting and start cooking.

Cheers!

And, of course, you've mastered measurements—in metrics as well as ounces and pounds. Just to jog your expertise, nevertheless, here are the weight equivalents again. For grams, which you're going to meet constantly, one way to help remember is to grasp that each ounce is approximately 28⅓ grams. You're on your own in reviewing liters versus quarts and how many whatevers make up a tablespoon.

1 pound (16 ounces)	453.6 grams
1 ounce	28.35 grams
3½ ounces	100 grams

MEASUREMENT GUIDE
FLUID WEIGHT

3 teaspoons =	1 tablespoon =	½ fluid ounce =	15 milliliters
4 tablespoons =	¼ cup =	2 fluid ounces =	60 milliliters
16 tablespoons =	1 cup =	8 fluid ounces =	240 milliliters
2 pints =	1 quart =	32 fluid ounces =	960 milliliters
4 quarts =	1 gallon =	128 fluid ounces =	3.8 liters
2 tablespoons =	1 ounce =	⅛ cup =	28 grams

DRY WEIGHT

Many people get confused when using cups to measure dry weight. As a rule of thumb, dry foods weigh half what liquids weigh, or:

4 tablespoons = ¼ cup = 1 dry ounce = 60 milliliters = 28 grams

ITEM NO.	FOODS, APPROXIMATE MEASURES, UNITS, AND WEIGHT (EDIBLE PART UNLESS FOOTNOTES INDICATE OTHERWISE)	CALORIES

DAIRY PRODUCTS (CHEESE, CREAM, IMITATION CREAM, MILK; RELATED PRODUCTS)

	Butter. See Fats, oils;	
	related products, items 103–108	
	Cheese:	
	Natural:	
1	Blue: 1 oz	100

ITEM NO.	FOODS, APPROXIMATE MEASURES, UNITS, AND WEIGHT (EDIBLE PART UNLESS FOOTNOTES INDICATE OTHERWISE)	CALORIES
2	Camembert (3 wedges per 4-oz container). 1 wedge	115
	Cheddar:	
3	Cut pieces: 1 oz	115
4	1 cubic inch	70
5	Shredded: 1 cup	455
	Cottage (curd, not pressed down):	
	Creamed (cottage cheese, 4% fat):	
6	Large curd: 1 cup	235
7	Small curd: 1 cup	220
8	Low fat (2%): 1 cup	205
9	Low fat (1%): 1 cup	165
10	Uncreamed (cottage cheese dry curd, less than ½% fat): 1 cup	125
11	Cream: 1 oz	100
	Mozzarella, made with—	
12	Whole milk: 1 oz	90
13	Part skim milk: 1 oz	80
	Parmesan, grated:	
14	Cup, not pressed down: 1 cup	455
15	Tablespoon: 1 tbsp	25
16	Ounce: 1 oz	130
17	Provolone: 1 oz	100
	Ricotta, made with—	
18	Whole milk: 1 cup	430
19	Part skim milk: 1 cup	340
20	Romano: 1 oz.	110
21	Swiss: 1 oz	105
	Pasteurized process cheese:	
22	American: 1 oz	105
23	Swiss: 1 oz	95
24	Pasteurized process cheese food, American. 1 oz	95
25	Pasteurized process cheese spread, American. 1 oz	80
	Cream, sweet:	
26	Half-and-half (cream and milk): 1 cup	315
27	1 tbsp	20
28	Light, coffee, or table: 1 cup	470
29	1 tbsp	30
	Whipping, unwhipped (volume about double when whipped):	

ITEM NO.	FOODS, APPROXIMATE MEASURES, UNITS, AND WEIGHT (EDIBLE PART UNLESS FOOTNOTES INDICATE OTHERWISE)	CALORIES
30	Light: 1 cup	700
31	1 tbsp	45
32	Heavy: 1 cup	820
33	1 tbsp	80
34	Whipped topping, (pressurized): 1 cup	155
35	1 tbsp	10
36	Cream, sour: 1 cup	495
37	1 tbsp	25
	Cream products, imitation (made with vegetable fat):	
	Sweet:	
	Creamers:	
38	Liquid (frozen): 1 cup	335
39	1 tbsp	20
40	Powdered: 1 cup	515
41	1 tsp	10
	Whipped topping:	
42	Frozen: 1 cup	240
43	1 tbsp	15
44	Powdered, made with whole milk. 1 cup	150
45	1 tbsp	10
46	Pressurized: 1 cup	185
47	1 tbsp	10
48	Sour dressing (imitation sour cream) made with nonfat dry milk. 1 cup	415
49	1 tbsp	20
	Ice cream. See Milk desserts, frozen (items 75–80).	
	Ice milk. See Milk desserts, frozen (items 81–83).	
	Milk:	
	Fluid:	
50	Whole (3.3% fat): 1 cup	150
	Lowfat 2%):	
51	No milk solids added: 1 cup	120
52	Milk solids added: Label claim less than 10 g of protein per cup. 1 cup	125
53	Label claim 10 or more grams of protein per cup (protein fortified). 1 cup	135
	Lowfat (1%):	
54	No milk solids added: 1 cup	100
	Milk solids added:	
55	Label claim less than 10 g of protein per cup. 1 cup	105

ITEM NO.	FOODS, APPROXIMATE MEASURES, UNITS, AND WEIGHT (EDIBLE PART UNLESS FOOTNOTES INDICATE OTHERWISE)	CALORIES
56	Label claim 10 or more grams of protein per cup (protein fortified). 1 cup	120
	Nonfat (skim):	
57	No milk solids added: 1 cup	85
	Milk solids added:	
58	Label claim less than 10 g of protein per cup. 1 cup	90
59	Label claim 10 or more grams of protein per cup (protein fortified). 1 cup	100
60	Buttermilk: 1 cup	100
	Canned:	
	Evaporated, unsweetened:	
61	Whole milk: 1 cup	340
62	Skim milk: 1 cup	200
63	Sweetened, condensed: 1 cup	980
	Dried:	
64	Buttermilk: 1 cup	465
	Nonfat instant:	
65	Envelope, net wt., 3.2 oz:[1] 1 envelope	325
66	Cup[2]: 1 cup	245
	Milk beverages:	
	Chocolate milk (commercial):	
67	Regular: 1 cup	210
68	Lowfat (2%): 1 cup	180
69	Lowfat (1%): 1 cup	160
70	Eggnog (commercial): 1 cup	340
	Malted milk, home-prepared with 1 cup of whole milk and 2 to 3 heaping tsp of malted milk powder (about ¾ oz):	
71	Chocolate: 1 cup of milk plus ¾ oz of powder.	235
72	Natural: 1 cup of milk plus ¾ oz of powder.	235
	Shakes, thick:[3]	
73	Chocolate, container, net wt., 10.6 oz. 1 container	355
74	Vanilla, container, net wt., 11 oz. 1 container	350
	Milk desserts, frozen:	
	Ice cream:	
	Regular (about 11% fat):	
75	Hardened: ½ gal	2,155
76	1 cup	270
77	3-fl oz container	100

ITEM NO.	FOODS, APPROXIMATE MEASURES, UNITS, AND WEIGHT (EDIBLE PART UNLESS FOOTNOTES INDICATE OTHERWISE)	CALORIES
78	Soft serve (frozen custard) 1 cup	375
79	Rich (about 16% fat), hardened. ½ gal	2,805
80	1 cup	350
	Ice milk:	
81	Hardened (about 4.3% fat): ½ gal	1,470
82	1 cup	185
83	Soft serve (about 2.6% fat): 1 cup	225
84	Sherbet (about 2% fat): ½ gal	2,160
85	1 cup	270
	Milk desserts, other:	
86	Custard, baked: 1 cup	305
	Puddings:	
	From home recipe:	
	Starch base:	
87	Chocolate: 1 cup	385
88	Vanilla (blancmange): 1 cup	285
89	Tapioca cream: 1 cup	220
	From mix (chocolate) and milk:	
90	Regular (cooked): 1 cup	320
91	Instant: 1 cup	325
	Yogurt:	
	With added milk solids:	
	Made with lowfat milk:	
92	Fruit-flavored:[4] 1 container, net wt., 8 oz	230
93	Plain: 1 container, net wt., 8 oz	145
94	Made with nonfat milk: 1 container, net wt., 8 oz	125
	Without added milk solids:	
95	Made with whole milk: 1 container, net wt., 8 oz.	140

EGGS

	Eggs, large (24 oz per dozen):	
	Raw:	
96	Whole, without shell: 1 egg	80
97	White: 1 white	15
98	Yolk: 1 yolk	65
	Cooked:	
99	Fried in butter: 1 egg	85
100	Hard-cooked, shell removed: 1 egg	80
101	Poached: 1 egg	80

ITEM NO.	FOODS, APPROXIMATE MEASURES, UNITS, AND WEIGHT (EDIBLE PART UNLESS FOOTNOTES INDICATE OTHERWISE)	CALORIES
102	Scrambled (milk added) in butter. Also omelet. 1 egg	95

FATS, OILS; RELATED PRODUCTS

Butter:
   Regular (1 brick or 4 sticks per lb):

103	Stick (½ cup): 1 stick	815
104	Tablespoon (about ⅛ stick). 1 tbsp	100
105	Pat (1 in square, ⅓ in high; 90 per lb). 1 pat	35
	Whipped (6 sticks or two 8-oz containers per lb).	
106	Stick (½ cup): 1 stick	540
107	Tablespoon (about ⅛ stick). 1 tbsp	65
108	Pat (1 ¼ in square, ⅓ in high; 120 per lb). 1 pat	25
109	Fats, cooking (vegetable shortenings). 1 cup	1,770
110	1 tbsp	110
111	Lard: 1 cup	1,850
112	1 tbsp	115
	Margarine:	
	Regular (1 brick or 4 sticks per lb):	
113	Stick (½ cup): 1 stick	815
114	Tablespoon (about ⅛ stick): 1 tbsp	100
115	Pat (1 in square, ⅓ in high; 90 per lb). 1 pat	35
116	Soft, two 8-oz containers per lb. 1 container	1,630
117	1 tbsp	100
	Whipped (6 sticks per lb):	
118	Stick (½ cup): 1 stick	545
119	Tablespoon (about ⅛ stick): 1 tbsp	70
	Oils, salad or cooking:	
120	Corn: 1 cup	1,925
121	1 tbsp	120
122	Olive: 1 cup	1,910
123	1 tbsp	120
124	Peanut: 1 cup	1,910
125	1 tbsp	120
126	Safflower: 1 cup	1,925
127	1 tbsp	120
128	Soybean oil, hydrogenated (partially hardened). 1 cup	1,925
129	1 tbsp	120
130	Soybean-cottonseed oil blend, hydrogenated. 1 cup	1,925

ITEM NO.	FOODS, APPROXIMATE MEASURES, UNITS, AND WEIGHT (EDIBLE PART UNLESS FOOTNOTES INDICATE OTHERWISE)	CALORIES
131	— 1 tbsp	120
	Salad dressings:	
	Commercial:	
	Blue cheese:	
132	Regular: 1 tbsp	75
133	Low calorie (5 Cal per tsp): 1 tbsp	15
	French:	
134	Regular: 1 tbsp	65
135	Low calorie (5 Cal per tsp): 1 tbsp	15
	Italian:	
136	Regular: 1 tbsp	85
137	Low calorie (2 Cal per tsp): 1 tbsp	10
138	Mayonnaise: 1 tbsp	100
	Mayonnaise type:	
139	Regular: 1 tbsp	65
140	Low calorie (8 Cal per tsp): 1 tbsp	20
141	Tartar sauce, regular: 1 tbsp	75
	Thousand Island:	
142	Regular: 1 tbsp	80
143	Low calorie (10 Cal per tsp): 1 tbsp	25
	From home recipe:	
144	Cooked type:[4] 1 tbsp	25

FISH, SHELLFISH, MEAT, POULTRY; RELATED PRODUCTS

	Fish and shellfish:	
145	Bluefish, baked with butter or margarine. 3 oz	135
	Clams:	
146	Raw, meat only: 3 oz	65
147	Canned, solids and liquid: 3 oz	45
148	Crabmeat (white or king), canned, not pressed down. 1 cup	135
149	Fish sticks, breaded, cooked, frozen (stick, 4 by 1 by ½ in). 1 fish stick or 1 oz	50
150	Haddock, breaded, fried:[5] 3 oz	140
151	Ocean perch, breaded, fried:[5] 1 fillet	195
152	Oysters, raw, meat only (13–19 medium Selects). 1 cup	160
153	Salmon, pink, canned, solids and liquid. 3 oz	120

ITEM NO.	FOODS, APPROXIMATE MEASURES, UNITS, AND WEIGHT (EDIBLE PART UNLESS FOOTNOTES INDICATE OTHERWISE)	CALORIES
154	Sardines, Atlantic, canned in oil, drained solids. 3 oz	175
155	Scallops, frozen, breaded, fried, reheated. 6 scallops	175
156	Shad, baked with butter or margarine, bacon. 3 oz	170
	Shrimp:	
157	Canned meat: 3 oz	100
158	French fried:[6] 3 oz	190
159	Tuna, canned in oil, drained solids. 3 oz	170
160	Tuna salad:[7] 1 cup	350
	Meat and meat products:	
161	Bacon (20 slices per lb, raw), broiled or fried, crisp. 2 slices	85
	Beef,[8] cooked:	
	Cuts braised, simmered or pot roasted:	
162	Lean and fat (piece, 2½ by 2½ by ¾ in). 3 oz	245
163	Lean only from item 162: 2.5 oz	140
	Ground beef, broiled:	
164	Lean with 10% fat: 3 oz or patty 3 by ⅝ in	185
165	Lean with 21% fat: 2.9 oz or patty 3 by ⅝ in	235
	Roast, oven cooked, no liquid added:	
	Relatively fat, such as rib:	
166	Lean and fat (2 pieces, 4⅛ by 2¼ by ¼ in). 3 oz	375
167	Lean only from item 166: 1.8 oz	125
	Relatively lean, such as heel of round:	
168	Lean and fat (2 pieces, 4⅛ by 2¼ by ¼ in). 3 oz	165
169	Lean only from item 168: 2.8 oz	125
	Steak:	
	Relatively fat–sirloin, broiled:	
170	Lean and fat (piece, 2½ by 2½ by ¾ in). 3 oz	330
171	Lean only from item 170: 2.0 oz	115
	Relatively lean–round, braised:	
172	Lean and fat (piece, 4⅛ by 2¼ by ½ in). 3 oz	220
173	Lean only from item 172: 2.4 oz	130
	Beef, canned:	
174	Corned beef: 3 oz	185
175	Corned beef hash: 1 cup	400
176	Beef, dried, chipped: 2½-oz jar	145
177	Beef and vegetable stew: 1 cup	220

ITEM NO.	FOODS, APPROXIMATE MEASURES, UNITS, AND WEIGHT (EDIBLE PART UNLESS FOOTNOTES INDICATE OTHERWISE)	CALORIES
178	Beef potpie (home recipe), baked[9] (piece, ⅓ of 9-in diam. pie). 1 piece	515
179	Chili con carne with beans, canned. 1 cup	340
180	Chop suey with beef and pork (home recipe). 1 cup	300
181	Heart, beef, lean, braised: 3 oz	160
	Lamb, cooked:	
	Chop, rib (cut 3 per lb with bone), broiled:	
182	Lean and fat: 3.1 oz	360
183	Lean only from item 182: 2 oz	120
	Leg, roasted:	
184	Lean and fat (2 pieces 4⅛ by 2¼ by ¼ in). 3 oz	235
185	Lean only from item 184: 2.5 oz	130
	Shoulder, roasted:	
186	Lean and fat (3 pieces, 2½ by 2½ by ¼ in). 3 oz	285
187	Lean only from item 186: 2.3 oz	130
188	Liver, beef, fried[10] (slice, 6½ by 2⅜ by ⅜ in). 3 oz	195
	Pork, cured, cooked:	
189	Ham, light cure, lean and fat, roasted (2 pieces, 4⅛ by 2¼ by ¼ in):[11] 3 oz	245
	Luncheon meat:	
190	Boiled ham, slice (8 per 8-oz pkg.). 1 oz	65
	Canned, spiced or unspiced:	
191	Slice, approx. 3 by 2 by ½ in. 1 slice	175
	Pork, fresh,[8] cooked:	
	Chop, loin (cut 3 per lb with bone), broiled:	
192	Lean and fat: 2.7 oz	305
193	Lean only from item 192: 2 oz	150
	Roast, oven cooked, no liquid added:	
194	Lean and fat (piece, 2½ by 2½ by ¾ in). 3 oz	310
195	Lean only from item 194: 2.4 oz	175
	Shoulder cut, simmered:	
196	Lean and fat (3 pieces, 2½ by 2½ by ¼ in). 3 oz	320
197	Lean only from item 196: 2.2 oz	135
	Sausages (see also Luncheon meat (items 190–191):	
198	Bologna, slice (8 per 8-oz pkg.). 1 slice	85
199	Braunschweiger, slice (6 per 6-oz pkg.). 1 slice	90
200	Brown and serve (10–11 per 8-oz pkg.), browned. 1 link	70
201	Deviled ham, canned: 1 tbsp	45
202	Frankfurter (8 per 1-lb pkg.), cooked (reheated). 1 frankfurter	170

ITEM NO.	FOODS, APPROXIMATE MEASURES, UNITS, AND WEIGHT (EDIBLE PART UNLESS FOOTNOTES INDICATE OTHERWISE)	CALORIES
203	Meat, potted (beef, chicken, turkey), canned. 1 tbsp	30
204	Pork link (16 per 1-lb pkg.), cooked. 1 link	60
	Salami:	
205	Dry type, slice (12 per 4-oz pkg.). 1 slice	45
206	Cooked type, slice (8 per 8-oz pkg.). 1 slice	90
207	Vienna sausage (7 per 4-oz can). 1 sausage	40
	Veal, medium fat, cooked, bone removed:	
208	Cutlet (4⅛ by 2¼ by ½ in), braised or broiled. 3 oz	185
209	Rib (2 pieces, 4⅛ by 2¼ by ¼ in), roasted. 3 oz	230
	Poultry and poultry products:	
	Chicken, cooked:	
210	Breast, fried,[12] bones removed, ½ breast (3.3 oz with bones). 2.8 oz	160
211	Drumstick, fried,[12] bones removed (2 oz with bones). 1.3 oz	90
212	Half broiler, broiled, bones removed (10.4 oz with bones). 6.3 oz	240
213	Chicken, canned, boneless: 3 oz	170
214	Chicken a la king, cooked (home recipe). 1 cup	470
215	Chicken and noodles, cooked (home recipe). 1 cup	365
	Chicken chow mein:	
216	Canned: 1 cup	95
217	From home recipe: 1 cup	255
218	Chicken potpie (home recipe), baked,[9] piece (⅓ of 9-in diam. pie). 1 piece	545
	Turkey, roasted, flesh without skin:	
219	Dark meat, piece, 2½ by 1⅝ by ¼ in. 4 pieces	175
220	Light meat, piece, 4 by 2 by ¼ in. 2 pieces	150
	Light and dark meat:	
221	Chopped or diced: 1 cup	265
222	Pieces (1 slice white meat, 4 by 2 by ¼ in with 2 slices dark meat 2½ by 1⅝ by ¼ in). 3 pieces	160

FRUITS AND FRUIT PRODUCTS

	Apples, raw, unpeeled, without cores:	
223	2¾-in diam. (about 3 per lb with cores). 1 apple	80
224	3¼ in diam. (about 2 per lb with cores). 1 apple	125

ITEM NO.	FOODS, APPROXIMATE MEASURES, UNITS, AND WEIGHT (EDIBLE PART UNLESS FOOTNOTES INDICATE OTHERWISE)	CALORIES
225	Applejuice, bottled or canned:[13] 1 cup	120
	Applesauce, canned:	
226	Sweetened: 1 cup	230
227	Unsweetened: 1 cup	100
	Apricots:	
228	Raw, without pits (about 12 per lb with pits). 3 apricots	55
229	Canned in heavy syrup (halves and syrup). 1 cup	220
	Dried:	
230	Uncooked (28 large or 37 medium halves per cup). 1 cup	340
231	Cooked, unsweetened, fruit and liquid. 1 cup	215
232	Apricot nectar, canned: 1 cup	145
	Avocados, raw, whole, without skins and seeds:	
233	California, mid- and late-winter (with skin and seed, 3⅛-in diam.; wt., 10 oz). 1 avocado	370
234	Florida, late summer and fall (with skin and seed, 3⅝-in diam.; wt., 1 lb). 1 avocado	390
235	Banana without peel (about 2.6 per lb with peel). 1 banana	100
236	Banana flakes: 1 tbsp	20
237	Blackberries, raw: 1 cup	85
238	Blueberries, raw: 1 cup	90
	Cantaloupe See Muskmelons (item 271)	
	Cherries:	
239	Sour (tart), red, pitted, canned, water pack. 1 cup	105
240	Sweet, raw, without pits and stems. 10 cherries	45
241	Cranberry juice cocktail, bottled, sweetened. 1 cup	165
242	Cranberry sauce, sweetened, canned, strained. 1 cup	405
	Dates:	
243	Whole, without pits: 10 dates	220
244	Chopped: 1 cup	490
245	Fruit cocktail, canned, in heavy syrup. 1 cup	195
	Grapefruit:	
	Raw, medium, 3¾-in diam. (about 1 lb 1 oz):	
246	Pink or red: ½ grapefruit with peel	50
247	White: ½ grapefruit with peel	45
248	Canned, sections with syrup: 1 cup	180
	Grapefruit juice:	
249	Raw, pink, red, or white: 1 cup	95
	Canned, white:	

ITEM NO.	FOODS, APPROXIMATE MEASURES, UNITS, AND WEIGHT (EDIBLE PART UNLESS FOOTNOTES INDICATE OTHERWISE)	CALORIES
250	Unsweetened: 1 cup	100
251	Sweetened: 1 cup	135
	Frozen, concentrate, unsweetened:	
252	Undiluted, 6-fl oz can: 1 can	300
253	Diluted with 3 parts water by volume. 1 cup	100
254	Dehydrated crystals, prepared with water (1 lb yields about 1 gal.) 1 cup	100
	Grapes, European type (adherent skin), raw:	
255	Thompson Seedless: 10 grapes	35
256	Tokay and Emperor, seeded types: 10 grapes[14]	40
	Grapejuice:	
257	Canned or bottled: 1 cup	165
	Frozen concentrate, sweetened:	
258	Undiluted, 6-fl oz can: 1 can	395
259	Diluted with 3 parts water by volume. 1 cup	135
260	Grape drink, canned: 1 cup	135
261	Lemon, raw, size 165, without peel and seeds (about 4 per lb with peels and seeds). 1 lemon	20
	Lemon juice:	
262	Raw: 1 cup	60
263	Canned, or bottled, unsweetened: 1 cup	55
264	Frozen, single strength, unsweetened, 6-fl oz can. 1 can	40
	Lemonade concentrate, frozen:	
265	Undiluted, 6-fl oz can: 1 can	425
266	Diluted with 4⅓ parts water by volume. 1 cup	105
	Limeade concentrate, frozen:	
267	Undiluted, 6-fl oz can: 1 can	410
268	Diluted with 4⅓ parts water by volume. 1 cup	100
	Limejuice:	
269	Raw: 1 cup	65
270	Canned, unsweetened: 1 cup	65
	Muskmelons, raw, with rind, without seed cavity:	
271	Cantaloupe, orange-fleshed (with rind and seed cavity, 5-in diam., 2⅓ lb). ½ melon with rind	80
272	Honeydew (with rind and seed cavity, 6½-in diam., 5¼ lb). 1/10 melon with rind	50
	Oranges, all commercial varieties, raw:	
273	Whole, 2⅝-in diam., without peel and seeds (about 2½ per lb with peel and seeds). 1 orange	65
274	Sections without membranes: 1 cup	90

ITEM NO.	FOODS, APPROXIMATE MEASURES, UNITS, AND WEIGHT (EDIBLE PART UNLESS FOOTNOTES INDICATE OTHERWISE)	CALORIES
	Orange juice:	
275	Raw, all varieties: 1 cup	110
276	Canned, unsweetened: 1 cup	120
	Frozen concentrate:	
277	Undiluted, 6-fl oz can: 1 can	360
278	Diluted with 3 parts water by volume. 1 cup	120
279	Dehydrated crystals, prepared with water (1 lb yields about 1 gal). 1 cup	115
	Orange and grapefruit juice:	
	Frozen concentrate:	
280	Undiluted, 6-fl oz can: 1 can	330
281	Diluted with 3 parts water by volume. 1 cup	110
282	Papayas, raw, ½-in cubes: 1 cup	55
	Peaches:	
	Raw:	
283	Whole, 2½-in diam., peeled, pitted (about 4 per lb with peels and pits). 1 peach	40
284	Sliced: 1 cup	65
	Canned, yellow-fleshed, solids and liquid (halves or slices):	
285	Syrup pack: 1 cup	200
286	Water pack: 1 cup	75
	Dried:	
287	Uncooked: 1 cup	420
288	Cooked, unsweetened, halves and juice. 1 cup	205
	Frozen, sliced, sweetened:	
289	10-oz container: 1 container	250
290	Cup: 1 cup	220
	Pears:	
	Raw, with skin, cored:	
291	Bartlett, 2½-in diam. (about 2½ per lb with cores and stems). 1 pear	100
292	Bosc, 2½-in diam. (about 3 per lb with cores and stems). 1 pear	85
293	D'Anjou, 3-in diam. (about 2 per lb with cores and stems). 1 pear	120
294	Canned, solids and liquid, syrup pack, heavy (halves or slices). 1 cup	195
	Pineapple:	
295	Raw, diced: 1 cup	80
	Canned, heavy syrup pack, solids and liquid:	

ITEM NO.	FOODS, APPROXIMATE MEASURES, UNITS, AND WEIGHT (EDIBLE PART UNLESS FOOTNOTES INDICATE OTHERWISE)	CALORIES
296	Crushed, chunks, tidbits: 1 cup	190
	Slices and liquid:	
297	Large: 1 slice; 2¼ tbsp liquid.	80
298	Medium: 1 slice; 1¼ tbsp liquid.	45
299	Pineapple juice, unsweetened, canned. 1 cup	140
	Plums:	
	Raw, without pits:	
300	Japanese and hybrid (2⅛-in diam., about 6½ per lb with pits). 1 plum	30
301	Prune-type (1½-in diam., about 15 per lb with pits). 1 plum	20
	Canned, heavy syrup pack (Italian prunes), with pits and liquid:	
302	Cup: 1 cup	215
303	Portion: 3 plums; 2¾ tbsp liquid.	110
	Prunes, dried, "softenized," with pits:	
304	Uncooked: 4 extra large or 5 large prunes.	110
305	Cooked, unsweetened, all sizes, fruit and liquid. 1 cup	255
306	Prune juice, canned or bottled: 1 cup	195
	Raisins, seedless:	
307	Cup, not pressed down: 1 cup	420
308	Packet, ½ oz (1½ tbsp): 1 packet	40
	Raspberries, red:	
309	Raw, capped, whole: 1 cup	70
310	Frozen, sweetened, 10-oz container: 1 container	280
	Rhubarb, cooked, added sugar:	
311	From raw: 1 cup	380
312	From frozen, sweetened: 1 cup	385
	Strawberries:	
313	Raw, whole berries, capped: 1 cup	55
	Frozen, sweetened:	
314	Sliced, 10-oz container: 1 container	310
315	Whole, 1-lb container (about 1¾ cups). 1 container	415
316	Tangerine, raw, 2⅜-in diam., size 176, without peel (about 4 per lb with peels and seeds). 1 tangerine	40
317	Tangerine juice, canned, sweetened. 1 cup	125
318	Watermelon, raw, 4 by 8 in wedge with rind and seeds (1/16 of 32⅔-lb melon, 10 by 16 in). 1 wedge with rind and seeds	110

ITEM   FOODS, APPROXIMATE MEASURES, UNITS, AND WEIGHT
NO.   (EDIBLE PART UNLESS FOOTNOTES INDICATE OTHERWISE) CALORIES

GRAIN PRODUCTS

	Bagel, 3-in diam.:	
319	Egg: 1 bagel	165
320	Water: 1 bagel	165
321	Barley, pearled, light, uncooked: 1 cup	700
	Biscuits, baking powder, 2-in diam. (enriched flour, vegetable shortening):	
322	From home recipe: 1 biscuit	105
323	From mix: 1 biscuit	90
	Breadcrumbs (enriched):[15]	
324	Dry, grated: 1 cup	390
	Soft. See White bread (items 339–350).	
	Breads:	
325	Boston brown bread, canned, slice 3¼ by ½ in.[15]	
	1 slice	95
	Cracked-wheat bread (¾ enriched wheat flour, ¼ cracked wheat):[15]	
326	Loaf, 1 lb: 1 loaf	1,195
327	Slice (18 per loaf): 1 slice	65
	French or vienna bread, enriched:[15]	
328	Loaf, 1 lb: 1 loaf	1,315
	Slice:	
329	French (5 by 2½ by 1 in): 1 slice	100
330	Vienna (4¾ by 4 by ½ in). 1 slice	75
	Italian bread, enriched:	
331	Loaf, 1 lb: 1 loaf	1,250
332	Slice, 4½ by 3¼ by ¾ in. 1 slice	85
	Raisin bread, enriched.[15]	
333	Loaf, 1 lb: 1 loaf	1,190
334	Slice (18 per loaf): 1 slice	65
	Rye bread:	
	American, light (⅔ enriched wheat flour, ⅓ rye flour):	
335	Loaf, 1 lb: 1 loaf	1,100
336	Slice (4¾ by 3¾ by ⁷⁄₁₆ in). 1 slice	60
	Pumpernickel (⅔ rye flour, ⅓ enriched wheat flour):	
337	Loaf, 1 lb: 1 loaf	1,115
338	Slice (5 by 4 by ⅜ in): 1 slice	80
	White bread, enriched:[15]	
	Soft-crumb type:	
339	Loaf, 1 lb: 1 loaf	1,225

ITEM NO.	FOODS, APPROXIMATE MEASURES, UNITS, AND WEIGHT (EDIBLE PART UNLESS FOOTNOTES INDICATE OTHERWISE)	CALORIES
340	Slice (18 per loaf): 1 slice	70
341	Slice, toasted: 1 slice	70
342	Slice (22 per loaf): 1 slice	55
343	Slice, toasted: 1 slice	55
344	Loaf, 1½ lb: 1 loaf	1,835
345	Slice (24 per loaf): 1 slice	75
346	Slice, toasted: 1 slice	75
347	Slice (28 per loaf): 1 slice	65
348	Slice toasted: 1 slice	65
349	Cubes: 1 cup	80
350	Crumbs: 1 cup	120
	Firm-crumb type:	
351	Loaf, 1 lb: 1 loaf	1,245
352	Slice (20 per loaf): 1 slice	65
353	Slice, toasted: 1 slice	65
354	Loaf, 2 lb: 1 loaf	2,495
355	Slice (34 per loaf): 1 slice	75
356	Slice, toasted: 1 slice	75
	Whole-wheat bread:	
	Soft-crumb type:[15]	
357	Loaf, 1 lb: 1 loaf	1,095
358	Slice (16 per loaf): 1 slice	65
359	Slice, toasted: 1 slice	65
	Firm-crumb type:[15]	
360	Loaf, 1 lb: 1 loaf	1,100
361	Slice (18 per loaf): 1 slice	60
362	Slice, toasted: 1 slice	60
	Breakfast cereals:	
	Hot type, cooked:	
	Corn (hominy) grits, degermed:	
363	Enriched: 1 cup	125
364	Unenriched: 1 cup	125
365	Farina, quick-cooking, enriched. 1 cup	105
366	Oatmeal or rolled oats: 1 cup	130
367	Wheat, rolled: 1 cup	180
368	Wheat, whole-meal: 1 cup	110
	Ready-to-eat:	
369	Bran flakes (40% bran), added sugar, salt, iron, vitamins. 1 cup	105
370	Bran flakes with raisins, added sugar, salt, iron, vitamins. 1 cup	145

ITEM NO.	FOODS, APPROXIMATE MEASURES, UNITS, AND WEIGHT (EDIBLE PART UNLESS FOOTNOTES INDICATE OTHERWISE)	CALORIES
	Corn flakes:	
371	Plain, added sugar, salt, iron, vitamins. 1 cup	95
372	Sugar-coated, added salt, iron, vitamins. 1 cup	155
373	Corn, oat flour, puffed, added sugar, salt, iron, vitamins. 1 cup	80
374	Corn, shredded, added sugar, salt, iron, thiamin, niacin. 1 cup	95
375	Oats, puffed, added sugar, salt, minerals, vitamins. 1 cup	100
	Rice, puffed:	
376	Plain, added iron, thiamin, niacin. 1 cup	60
377	Presweetened, added salt, iron, vitamins. 1 cup	115
378	Wheat flakes, added sugar, salt, iron, vitamins. 1 cup	105
	Wheat, puffed:	
379	Plain, added iron, thiamin, niacin. 1 cup	55
380	Presweetened, added salt, iron, vitamins. 1 cup	140
381	Wheat, shredded, plain: 1 oblong biscuit or ½ cup spoon-size biscuits.	90
382	Wheat germ, without salt and sugar, toasted. 1 tbsp	25
383	Buckwheat flour, light, sifted: 1 cup	340
384	Bulgur, canned, seasoned: 1 cup	245
	Cake icings. See Sugars and Sweets (items 532–536).	
	Cakes made from cake mixes with enriched flour:[16]	
	Angelfood:	
385	Whole caked (9¾-in diam. tube cake). 1 cake	1,645
386	Piece, 1/12 of cake: 1 piece	135
	Coffeecake:	
387	Whole cake (7¾ by 5⅝ by 1¼ in). 1 cake	1,385
388	Piece, 1/6 of cake: 1 piece	230
	Cupcakes, made with egg, milk, 2½-in diam.:	
389	Without icing: 1 cupcake	90
390	With chocolate icing: 1 cupcake	130
	Devil's food with chocolate icing:	
391	Whole, 2 layer cake (8- or 9-in diam.). 1 cake	3,755
392	Piece, 1/16 of cake: 1 piece	235
393	Cupcake, 2½-in diam: 1 cupcake	120

ITEM NO.	FOODS, APPROXIMATE MEASURES, UNITS, AND WEIGHT (EDIBLE PART UNLESS FOOTNOTES INDICATE OTHERWISE)	CALORIES
	Gingerbread:	
394	Whole cake (8-in square): 1 cake	1,575
395	Piece, 1/9 of cake: 1 piece	175
	White, 2 layer with chocolate icing:	
396	Whole cake (8- or 9-in diam.): 1 cake	4,000
397	Piece, 1/16 of cake: 1 piece	250
	Yellow, 2 layer with chocolate icing:	
398	Whole cake (8- or 9-in diam.): 1 cake	3,735
399	Piece, 1/16 of cake: 1 piece	235
	Cakes made from home recipes using enriched flour:	
	Boston cream pie with custard filling:	
400	Whole cake (8-in. diam.): 1 cake	2,490
401	Piece, 1/12 of cake: 1 piece	210
	Fruitcake, dark:	
402	Loaf, 1-lb (7½ by 2 by 1½ in). 1 loaf	1,720
403	Slice, 1/30 of loaf: 1 slice	55
	Plain, sheet cake:	
	Without icing:	
404	Whole cake (8-in square): 1 cake	2,830
405	Piece, 1/9 of cake: 1 piece	315
	With uncooked white icing:	
406	Whole cake (9-in square): 1 cake	4,020
407	Piece, 1/9 of cake: 1 piece	445
	Pound:[17]	
408	Loaf, 8½ by 3½ by 3¼ in. 1 loaf	2,725
409	Slice, 1/17 of loaf: 1 slice	160
	Spongecake:	
410	Whole cake (9¾-in diam. tube cake). 1 cake	2,345
411	Piece, 1/12 of cake: 1 piece	195
	Cookies made with enriched flour:[18]	
	Brownies with nuts:	
	Home-prepared, 1¾ by 1¾ by ⅞ in:	
412	From home recipe: 1 brownie	95
413	From commercial recipe: 1 brownie	85
414	Frozen, with chocolate icing,[19] 1½ by 1¾ by ⅞ in. 1 brownie	105
	Chocolate chip:	
415	Commercial, 2¼-in diam., ⅜ in thick. 4 cookies	200
416	From home recipe, 2⅓-in diam. 4 cookies	205
417	Fig bars, square (1⅝ by 1⅝ by ⅜ in) or rectangular (1½ by 1¾ by ½ in). 4 cookies	200

ITEM NO.	FOODS, APPROXIMATE MEASURES, UNITS, AND WEIGHT (EDIBLE PART UNLESS FOOTNOTES INDICATE OTHERWISE)	CALORIES
418	Gingersnaps, 2-in diam., ¼ in thick. 4 cookies	90
419	Macaroons, 2¾-in diam., ¼ in thick. 2 cookies	180
420	Oatmeal with raisins, 2⅝-in diam., ¼ in thick. 4 cookies	235
421	Plain, prepared from commercial chilled dough, 2½-in diam., ¼ in thick. 4 cookies	240
422	Sandwich type (chocolate or vanilla), 1¾-in diam., ⅜ in thick. 4 cookies	200
423	Vanilla wafers, 1¾-in diam., ¼ in thick. 10 cookies	185
	Cornmeal:	
424	Whole-ground, unbolted, dry form. 1 cup	435
425	Bolted (nearly whole-grain), dry form. 1 cup	440
	Degermed, enriched:	
426	Dry form: 1 cup	500
427	Cooked: 1 cup	120
	Degermed, unenriched:	
428	Dry form: 1 cup	500
429	Cooked: 1 cup	120
	Crackers:[15]	
430	Graham, plain, 2½-in square: 2 crackers	55
431	Rye wafers, whole-grain, 1⅞ by 3½ in. 2 wafers	45
432	Saltines, made with enriched flour. 4 crackers or 1 packet	50
	Danish pastry (enriched flour), plain without fruit or nuts:[19]	
433	Packaged ring, 12 oz: 1 ring	1,435
434	Round piece, about 4¼-in diam. by 1 in. 1 pastry	275
435	Ounce: 1 oz	120
	Doughnuts, made with enriched flour:	
436	Cake type, plain, 2½-in diam., 1 in high. 1 doughnut	100
437	Yeast-leavened, glazed, 3¾-in diam., 1¼ in high. 1 doughnut	205
	Macaroni, enriched, cooked (cut lengths, elbows, shells):	
438	Firm stage (hot): 1 cup	190
	Tender stage:	
439	Cold macaroni: 1 cup	115
440	Hot macaroni: 1 cup	155
	Macaroni (enriched) and cheese:	
441	Canned:[20] 1 cup	230
442	From home recipe (served hot):[21] 1 cup	430

ITEM NO.	FOODS, APPROXIMATE MEASURES, UNITS, AND WEIGHT (EDIBLE PART UNLESS FOOTNOTES INDICATE OTHERWISE)	CALORIES
	Muffins made with enriched flour:[15]	
	From home recipe:	
443	Blueberry, 2⅜-in diam., 1½ in high. 1 muffin	110
444	Bran: 1 muffin	105
445	Corn (enriched degermed cornmeal and flour), 2⅜-in diam., 1½ in high. 1 muffin	125
446	Plain, 3-in diam., 1½ in high. 1 muffin	120
	From mix, egg, milk:	
447	Corn, 2⅜-in diam., 1½ in high:[22] 1 muffin	130
448	Noodles (egg noodles), enriched, cooked. 1 cup	200
449	Noodles, chow mein, canned: 1 cup	220
	Pancakes, (4-in diam.):[15]	
450	Buckwheat, made from mix (with buckwheat and enriched flours), egg and milk added. 1 cake	55
	Plain:	
451	Made from home recipe using enriched flour. 1 cake	60
452	Made from mix with enriched flour, egg and milk added. 1 cake	60
	Pies, piecrust made with enriched flour, vegetable shortening (9-in diam.):	
	Apple:	
453	Whole: 1 pie	2,420
454	Sector, ⅐ of pie: 1 sector	345
	Banana cream:	
455	Whole: 1 pie	2,010
456	Sector, ⅐ of pie: 1 sector	285
	Blueberry:	
457	Whole: 1 pie	2,285
458	Sector, ⅐ of pie: 1 sector	325
	Cherry:	
459	Whole: 1 pie	2,465
460	Sector, ⅐ of pie: 1 sector	350
	Custard:	
461	Whole: 1 pie	1,985
462	Sector, ⅐ of pie: 1 sector	285
	Lemon meringue:	
463	Whole: 1 pie	2,140
464	Sector, ⅐ of pie: 1 sector	305
	Mince:	
465	Whole: 1 pie	2,560

ITEM NO.	FOODS, APPROXIMATE MEASURES, UNITS, AND WEIGHT (EDIBLE PART UNLESS FOOTNOTES INDICATE OTHERWISE)	CALORIES
466	Sector, 1/7 of pie: 1 sector	365
	Peach:	
467	Whole: 1 pie	2,410
468	Sector, 1/7 of pie: 1 sector	345
	Pecan:	
469	Whole: 1 pie	3,450
470	Sector, 1/7 of pie: 1 sector	495
	Pumpkin:	
471	Whole: 1 pie	1,920
472	Sector, 1/7 of pie: 1 sector	275
473	Piecrust (home recipe) made with enriched flour and vegetable shortening, baked. 1 pie shell, 9-in diam.	900
474	Piecrust mix with enriched flour and vegetable shortening, 10-oz pkg. prepared and baked. Piecrust for 2-crust pie, 9-in diam.	1,485
475	Pizza (cheese), baked, 4¾-in sector; ⅛ of 12-in diam. pie:[9] 1 sector	145
	Popcorn, popped:	
476	Plain, large kernel: 1 cup	25
477	With oil (coconut) and salt added, large kernel. 1 cup	40
478	Sugar coated: 1 cup	135
	Pretzels, made with enriched flour:	
479	Dutch, twisted, 2¾ by 2⅝ in. 1 pretzel	60
480	Thin, twisted, 3¼ by 2¼ by ¼ in. 10 pretzels	235
481	Stick, 2¼ in long: 10 pretzels	10
	Rice, white, enriched:	
482	Instant, ready-to-serve, hot: 1 cup	180
	Long grain:	
483	Raw: 1 cup	670
484	Cooked, served hot: 1 cup	225
	Parboiled:	
485	Raw: 1 cup	685
486	Cooked, served hot: 1 cup	185
	Rolls, enriched:[15]	
	Commercial:	
487	Brown-and-serve (12 per 12-oz pkg.), browned. 1 roll	85
488	Cloverleaf or pan, 2½-in diam., 2 in high. 1 roll	85

ITEM NO.	FOODS, APPROXIMATE MEASURES, UNITS, AND WEIGHT (EDIBLE PART UNLESS FOOTNOTES INDICATE OTHERWISE)	CALORIES
489	Frankfurter and hamburger (8 per 11½-oz pkg.). 1 roll	120
490	Hard, 3¾-in diam., 2 in high. 1 roll	155
491	Hoagie or submarine, 11½ by 3 by 2½ in. 1 roll	390
	From home recipe:	
492	Cloverleaf, 2½-in diam., 2 in high. 1 roll	120
	Spaghetti, enriched, cooked:	
493	Firm stage, "al dente," served hot. 1 cup	190
494	Tender stage, served hot. 1 cup	155
	Spaghetti (enriched) in tomato sauce with cheese:	
495	From home recipe: 1 cup	260
496	Canned: 1 cup	190
	Spaghetti (enriched) with meat balls and tomato sauce:	
497	From home recipe: 1 cup	330
498	Canned: 1 cup	260
499	Toaster pastries: 1 pastry	200
	Waffles, made with enriched flour, 7-in diam.:[15]	
500	From home recipe: 1 waffle	210
501	From mix, egg and milk added: 1 waffle	205
	Wheat flours:	
	All-purpose or family flour, enriched:	
502	Sifted, spooned: 1 cup	420
503	Unsifted, spooned: 1 cup	455
504	Cake or pastry flour, enriched, sifted, spooned. 1 cup	350
505	Self-rising, enriched, unsifted, spooned. 1 cup	440
506	Whole-wheat, from hard wheats, stirred. 1 cup	400

LEGUMES (DRY), NUTS, SEEDS; RELATED PRODUCTS

	Almonds, shelled:	
507	Chopped (about 130 almonds): 1 cup	775
508	Slivered, not pressed down (about 115 almonds). 1 cup	690
	Beans, dry:	
	Common varieties as Great Northern, navy, and others:	
	Cooked, drained:	
509	Great Northern: 1 cup	210
510	Pea (navy): 1 cup	225

ITEM NO.	FOODS, APPROXIMATE MEASURES, UNITS, AND WEIGHT (EDIBLE PART UNLESS FOOTNOTES INDICATE OTHERWISE)	CALORIES
	Canned, solids and liquid:	
	White with—	
511	Frankfurters (sliced): 1 cup	365
512	Pork and tomato sauce: 1 cup	310
513	Pork and sweet sauce: 1 cup	385
514	Red kidney: 1 cup	230
515	Lima, cooked, drained: 1 cup	260
516	Blackeye peas, dry, cooked (with residual cooking liquid). 1 cup	190
517	Brazil nuts, shelled (6–8 large kernels). 1 oz	185
518	Cashew nuts, roasted in oil: 1 cup	785
	Coconut meat, fresh:	
519	Piece, about 2 by 2 by ½ in: 1 piece	155
520	Shredded or grated, not pressed down. 1 cup	275
521	Filberts (hazelnuts), chopped (about 60 kernels). 1 cup	730
522	Lentils, whole, cooked: 1 cup	210
523	Peanuts, roasted in oil, salted (whole, halves, chopped). 1 cup	840
524	Peanut butter: 1 tbsp	95
525	Peas, split, dry, cooked: 1 cup	230
526	Pecans, chopped or pieces (about 120 large halves). 1 cup	810
527	Pumpkin and squash kernels, dry, hulled. 1 cup	775
528	Sunflower seeds, dry, hulled: 1 cup	810
	Walnuts:	
	Black:	
529	Chopped or broken kernels: 1 cup	785
530	Ground (finely): 1 cup	500
531	Persian or English, chopped (about 60 halves). 1 cup	780

SUGARS AND SWEETS

	Cake icings:	
	Boiled, white:	
532	Plain: 1 cup	295
533	With coconut: 1 cup	605
	Uncooked:	
534	Chocolate made with milk and butter. 1 cup	1,035

ITEM NO.	FOODS, APPROXIMATE MEASURES, UNITS, AND WEIGHT (EDIBLE PART UNLESS FOOTNOTES INDICATE OTHERWISE)	CALORIES
535	Creamy fudge from mix and water. 1 cup	830
536	White: 1 cup	1,200
	Candy:	
537	Caramels, plain or chocolate: 1 oz	115
	Chocolate:	
538	Milk, plain: 1 oz	145
539	Semisweet, small pieces (60 per oz). 1 cup or 6-oz pkg.	860
540	Chocolate-coated peanuts: 1 oz	160
541	Fondant, uncoated (mints, candy corn, other). 1 oz	105
542	Fudge, chocolate, plain: 1 oz	115
543	Gum drops: 1 oz	100
544	Hard: 1 oz	110
545	Marshmallows: 1 oz	90
	Chocolate-flavored beverage powders (about 4 heaping tsp per oz):	
546	With nonfat dry milk: 1 oz	100
547	Without milk: 1 oz	100
548	Honey, strained or extracted: 1 tbsp	65
549	Jams and preserves: 1 tbsp	55
550	1 packet	40
551	Jellies: 1 tbsp	50
552	1 packet	40
	Syrups:	
	Chocolate-flavored syrup or topping:	
553	Thin type: 1 fl oz or 2 tbsp	90
554	Fudge type: 1 fl oz or 2 tbsp	125
	Molasses, cane:	
555	Light (first extraction): 1 tbsp	50
556	Blackstrap (third extraction): 1 tbsp	45
557	Sorghum: 1 tbsp	55
558	Table blends, chiefly corn, light and dark. 1 tbsp	60
	Sugars:	
559	Brown, pressed down: 1 cup	820
	White:	
560	Granulated: 1 cup	770
561	1 tbsp	45
562	1 packet	23
563	Powdered, sifted, spooned into cup. 1 cup	385

VEGETABLES AND VEGETABLE PRODUCTS

	Asparagus, green:	
	Cooked, drained:	
	Cuts and tips, 1½- to 2-in lengths:	
564	From raw: 1 cup	30
565	From frozen: 1 cup	40
	Spears, ½-in diam. at base:	
566	From raw: 4 spears	10
567	From frozen: 4 spears	15
568	Canned, spears, ½-in diam. at base. 4 spears	15
	Beans;	
	Lima, immature seeds, frozen, cooked, drained:	
569	Thick-seeded types (Fordhooks): 1 cup	170
570	Thin-seeded types (baby limas): 1 cup	210
	Snap:	
	Green:	
	Cooked, drained:	
571	From raw (cuts and French style). 1 cup	30
	From frozen:	
572	Cuts: 1 cup	35
573	French style: 1 cup	35
574	Canned, drained solids (cuts). 1 cup	30
	Yellow or wax:	
	Cooked, drained:	
575	From raw (cuts and French style). 1 cup	30
576	From frozen (cuts): 1 cup	35
577	Canned, drained solids (cuts). 1 cup	30
	Beans, mature. See Beans, dry (items 509–515) and Blackeye peas, dry (item 516).	
	Bean sprouts (mung):	
578	Raw: 1 cup	35
579	Cooked, drained; 1 cup	35
	Beets:	
	Cooked, drained, peeled:	
580	Whole beets, 2-in diam. 2 beets	30
581	Diced or sliced: 1 cup	55
	Canned, drained solids:	
582	Whole beets, small: 1 cup	60
583	Diced or sliced: 1 cup	65

ITEM NO.	FOODS, APPROXIMATE MEASURES, UNITS, AND WEIGHT (EDIBLE PART UNLESS FOOTNOTES INDICATE OTHERWISE)	CALORIES
584	Beet greens, leaves and stems, cooked, drained. 1 cup	25
	Blackeye peas, immature seeds, cooked and drained:	
585	From raw: 1 cup	180
586	From frozen: 1 cup	220
	Broccoli, cooked, drained:	
	From raw:	
587	Stalk, medium size: 1 stalk	45
588	Stalks cut into ½-in pieces: 1 cup	40
	From frozen:	
589	Stalk, 4½ to 5 in long: 1 stalk	10
590	Chopped: 1 cup	50
	Brussels sprouts, cooked, drained:	
591	From raw, 7–8 sprouts (1¼- to 1½-in diam.). 1 cup	55
592	From frozen: 1 cup	50
	Cabbage:	
	Common varieties:	
	Raw:	
593	Coarsely shredded or sliced: 1 cup	15
594	Finely shredded or chopped: 1 cup	20
595	Cooked, drained: 1 cup	30
596	Red, raw, coarsely shredded or sliced. 1 cup	20
597	Savoy, raw, coarsely shredded or sliced. 1 cup	15
598	Cabbage, celery (also called pe-tsai or wongbok), raw, 1-in pieces. 1 cup	10
599	Cabbage, white mustard (also called bokchoy or pakchoy), cooked, drained. 1 cup	25
	Carrots:	
	Raw, without crowns and tips, scraped:	
600	Whole, 7½ by 1⅛ in, or strips, 2½ to 3 in long. 1 carrot or 18 strips	30
601	Grated: 1 cup	45
602	Cooked (crosswise cuts), drained: 1 cup	50
	Canned:	
603	Sliced, drained solids: 1 cup	45
604	Strained or junior (baby food): 1 oz (1¾ to 2 tbsp)	10
	Cauliflower:	
605	Raw, chopped: 1 cup	31
	Cooked, drained:	
606	From raw (flower buds): 1 cup	30

ITEM NO.	FOODS, APPROXIMATE MEASURES, UNITS, AND WEIGHT (EDIBLE PART UNLESS FOOTNOTES INDICATE OTHERWISE)	CALORIES
607	From frozen (flowerets): 1 cup	30
	Celery, Pascal type, raw:	
608	Stalk, large outer, 8 by 1½ in, at root end. 1 stalk	5
609	Pieces, diced: 1 cup	20
	Collards, cooked, drained:	
610	From raw (leaves without stems): 1 cup	65
611	From frozen (chopped): 1 cup	50
	Corn, sweet:	
	Cooked, drained:	
612	From raw, ear 5 by 1¾ in: 1 ear	70
	From frozen:	
613	Ear, 5 in long: 1 ear	120
614	Kernels: 1 cup	130
	Canned:	
615	Cream style: 1 cup	210
	Whole kernel:	
616	Vacuum pack: 1 cup	175
617	Wet pack, drained solids: 1 cup	140
	Cowpeas. See Blackeye peas.	
	(Items 585–586).	
	Cucumber slices, ⅛ in thick (large, 2⅛-in diam.; small, 1¾-in diam.):	
618	With peel: 6 large or 8 small slices	5
619	Without peel: 6½ large or 9 small pieces.	5
620	Dandelion greens, cooked, drained: 1 cup	35
621	Endive, curly (including escarole), raw, small pieces. 1 cup	10
	Kale, cooked, drained:	
622	From raw (leaves without stems and midribs): 1 cup	45
623	From frozen (leaf style): 1 cup	40
	Lettuce, raw:	
	Butterhead, as Boston types:	
624	Head, 5-in diam: 1 head	25
625	Leaves: 1 outer or 2 inner or 3 heart leaves.	Trace
	Crisphead, as Iceberg:	
626	Head, 6-in diam: 1 head	70
627	Wedge, ¼ of head: 1 wedge	20
628	Pieces, chopped or shredded: 1 cup	5
629	Looseleaf (bunching varieties including romaine or cos), chopped or shredded pieces. 1 cup	10

ITEM NO.	FOODS, APPROXIMATE MEASURES, UNITS, AND WEIGHT (EDIBLE PART UNLESS FOOTNOTES INDICATE OTHERWISE)	CALORIES
630	Mushrooms, raw, sliced or chopped: 1 cup	20
631	Mustard greens, without stems and midribs, cooked, drained. 1 cup	30
632	Okra pods, 3 by ⅝ in, cooked: 10 pods	30
	Onions:	
	Mature:	
	Raw:	
633	Chopped: 1 cup	65
634	Sliced: 1 cup	45
635	Cooked (whole or sliced), drained. 1 cup	60
636	Young green, bulb (⅜-in diam.) and white portion of top. 6 onions	15
637	Parsley, raw, chopped: 1 tbsp	Trace
638	Parsnips, cooked (diced or 2-in lengths). 1 cup	100
	Peas, green:	
	Canned:	
639	Whole, drained solids: 1 cup	150
640	Strained (baby food): 1 oz (1¾ to 2 tbsp)	15
641	Frozen, cooked, drained: 1 cup	110
642	Peppers, hot, red, without seeds, dried (ground chili powder, added seasonings). 1 tsp	5
	Peppers, sweet (about 5 per lb, whole), stem and seeds removed:	
643	Raw: 1 pod	15
644	Cooked, boiled, drained: 1 pod	15
	Potatoes, cooked:	
645	Baked, peeled after baking (about 2 per lb, raw). 1 potato	145
	Boiled (about 3 per lb, raw):	
646	Peeled after boiling: 1 potato	105
647	Peeled before boiling: 1 potato	90
	French-fried, strip, 2 to 3½ in long:	
648	Prepared from raw: 10 strips	135
649	Frozen, oven heated: 10 strips	110
650	Hashed brown, prepared from frozen. 1 cup	345
	Mashed, prepared from—	
	Raw:	
651	Milk added: 1 cup	135
652	Milk and butter added: 1 cup	195
653	Dehydrated flakes (without milk), water, milk, butter, and salt added. 1 cup	195

ITEM NO.	FOODS, APPROXIMATE MEASURES, UNITS, AND WEIGHT (EDIBLE PART UNLESS FOOTNOTES INDICATE OTHERWISE)	CALORIES
654	Potato chips, 1¾ by 2½ in oval cross section. 10 chips	115
655	Potato salad, made with cooked salad dressing. 1 cup	250
656	Pumpkin, canned: 1 cup	80
657	Radishes, raw (prepackaged) stem ends, rootlets cut off. 4 radishes	5
658	Sauerkraut, canned, solids and liquid. 1 cup	40
	Southern peas. See Blackeye peas (items 585–586).	
	Spinach:	
659	Raw, chopped: 1 cup	15
	Cooked, drained:	
660	From raw: 1 cup	40
	From frozen:	
661	Chopped: 1 cup	45
662	Leaf: 1 cup	45
663	Canned, drained solids: 1 cup	50
	Squash, cooked:	
664	Summer (all varieties), diced, drained. 1 cup	30
665	Winter (all varieties), baked, mashed. 1 cup	130
	Sweet potatoes:	
	Cooked (raw, 5 by 2 in; about 2½ per lb):	
666	Baked in skin, peeled: 1 potato	160
667	Boiled in skin, peeled: 1 potato	170
668	Candied, 2½ by 2-in piece: 1 piece	175
	Canned:	
669	Solid pack (mashed): 1 cup	275
670	Vacuum pack, piece 2¾ by 1 in. 1 piece	45
	Tomatoes:	
671	Raw, 2⅗-in diam. (3 per 12 oz pkg.). 1 tomato	25
672	Canned, solids and liquid: 1 cup	50
673	Tomato catsup: 1 cup	290
674	1 tbsp	15
	Tomato juice, canned:	
675	Cup: 1 cup	45
676	Glass (6 fl oz): 1 glass	35
677	Turnips, cooked, diced: 1 cup	35
	Turnip greens, cooked, drained:	
678	From raw (leaves and stems): 1 cup	30
679	From frozen (chopped): 1 cup	40
680	Vegetables, mixed, frozen, cooked: 1 cup	115

| ITEM | FOODS, APPROXIMATE MEASURES, UNITS, AND WEIGHT | |
| NO. | (EDIBLE PART UNLESS FOOTNOTES INDICATE OTHERWISE) | CALORIES |

MISCELLANEOUS ITEMS

	Baking powders for home use:	
	Sodium aluminum suflate:	
681	With monocalcium phosphate monohydrate. 1 tsp	5
682	With monocalcium phosphate monohydrate, calcium sulfate. 1 tsp	5
683	Straight phosphate: 1 tsp	5
684	Low sodium: 1 tsp	5
685	Barbecue sauce: 1 cup	230
	Beverages, alcoholic:	
686	Beer: 12 fl oz	150
	Gin, rum, vodka, whisky:	
687	80-proof: 1½-fl oz jigger	95
688	86-proof: 1½-fl oz jigger	105
689	90-proof: 1½-fl oz jigger	110
	Wines:	
690	Dessert: 3½-fl oz glass	140
691	Table: 3½-fl oz glass	85
	Beverages, carbonated, sweetened, nonalcoholic:	
692	Carbonated water: 12 fl oz	115
693	Cola type: 12 fl oz	145
694	Fruit-flavored sodas and Tom Collins mixer. 12 fl oz	170
695	Ginger ale: 12 fl oz	115
696	Root beer: 12 fl oz	150
	Chili powder. See Peppers, hot, red (item 642).	
	Chocolate:	
697	Bitter or baking: 1 oz	145
	Semisweet, see Candy, chocolate (item 539).	
698	Gelatin, dry: 1 7-g envelope	25
699	Gelatin dessert prepared with gelatin dessert powder and water. 1 cup	140
700	Mustard, prepared, yellow: 1 tsp or individual serving pouch or cup	5
	Olives, pickled, canned:	
701	Green: 4 medium or 3 extra large or 2 giant	15
702	Ripe, Mission: 3 small or 2 large	15
	Pickles, cucumber:	

ITEM NO.	FOODS, APPROXIMATE MEASURES, UNITS, AND WEIGHT (EDIBLE PART UNLESS FOOTNOTES INDICATE OTHERWISE)	CALORIES
703	Dill, medium, whole, 3¾ in long, 1¼-in diam. 1 pickle	5
704	Fresh-pack, slices 1½-in diam., ¼ in thick. 2 slices	10
705	Sweet, gherkin, small, whole, about 2½ in long, ¾-in diam. 1 pickle	20
706	Relish, finely chopped, sweet: 1 tbsp	20
	Popcorn. See items 476–478.	
707	Popsicle, 3-fl oz size: 1 popsicle	70
	Soups:	
	Canned, condensed:	
	Prepared with equal volume of milk:	
708	Cream of chicken: 1 cup	180
709	Cream of mushroom: 1 cup	215
710	Tomato: 1 cup	175
	Prepared with equal volume of water:	
711	Bean with pork: 1 cup	170
712	Beef broth, bouillon, consomme. 1 cup	30
713	Beef noodle: 1 cup	65
714	Clam chowder, Manhattan type (with tomatoes, without milk). 1 cup	80
715	Cream of chicken: 1 cup	95
716	Cream of mushroom: 1 cup	135
717	Minestrone: 1 cup	105
718	Split pea: 1 cup	145
719	Tomato: 1 cup	90
720	Vegetable beef: 1 cup	80
721	Vegetarian: 1 cup	80
	Dehydrated:	
722	Bouillon cube, ½ in: 1 cube	5
	Mixes:	
	Unprepared:	
723	Onion: 1½-oz pkg	150
	Prepared with water:	
724	Chicken noodle: 1 cup	55
725	Onion: 1 cup	35
726	Tomato vegetable with noodles. 1 cup	65
727	Vinegar, cider: 1 tbsp	Trace
728	White sauce, medium, with enriched flour. 1 cup	405
	Yeast:	
729	Baker's, dry, active: 1 pkg	20
730	Brewer's, dry: 1 tbsp	25

[1]Yields 1 qt of fluid milk when reconstituted according to package directions.

[2]Weight applies to product with label claim of 1⅓ cups equal 3.2 oz.

[3]Applies to products made from thick shake mixes and that do not contain added ice cream.

[4]Product made with regular-type margarine.

[5]Dipped in egg, milk or water, and bread crumbs; fried in vegetable shortening.

[6]Dipped in egg, bread crumbs, and flour or batter.

[7]Prepared with tuna, celery, salad dressing (mayonnaise type), pickle, onion, and egg.

[8]Outer layer of fat on the cut was removed to within approximately ½ in of the lean.

[9]Crust made with vegetable shortening and enriched flour.

[10]Regular-type margarine used.

[11]Value varies widely.

[12]Vegetable shortening used.

[13]Also applies to pasteurized apple cider.

[14]Weight includes seeds. Without seeds, weight of the edible portion is 57 g.

[15]Made with vegetable shortening.

[16]Value varies with the brand. Consult the label.

[17]Equal weights of flour, sugar, eggs, and vegetable shortening.

[18]Products are commercial unless otherwise specified.

[19]Icing made with butter.

[20]Made with corn oil.

[21]Made with regular margarine.

[22]Made with enriched degermed cornmeal and enriched flour.

Appendix: About the Recipes—and After the 21 Days

Many of the recipes in this book came from the Structure House menus. I fiddled around with some and turned southern Carolinian dishes to southern Italian dishes. Others I made up, and friends and relatives (even a few strangers) provided me with more. And there are some that have been in my files for years. I have no idea where they came from. I have prepared them all and have tried to include the ones I thought best for this diet.

Remember, after the 21-day period on 700 calories, you may then go to 1000 calories for a week. Don't be afraid of a slight weight gain. It is only the added sodium which is retaining the water in your body. *You are still losing weight!* The water *will* pass through your body. After a week on 1000 calories, you may go to 1200 calories. *You will still lose weight on that!* When you reach your goal, go onto the maintenance level, which is discussed more in the section on nutrition (Chapter 7). Check the calorie chart, choose wisely, and you can't go wrong.

Keep track of your progress using the following charts.

Don't forget that weight loss should be achieved gradually and that long term weight loss is achieved only through structured eating and good common sense.

The chart will help you to track your progress for the first six weeks of your new structured life.

In week six, you'll be eating 1800 calories per day, which, for most people, is still below maintenance level. You'll still be losing weight. Remember the formula for determining the calorie level that will maintain your desired weight:

men: desired weight × 15 = maintenance level
women: desired weight × 12 = maintenance level

This formula is based upon moderate physical activity.

700 Calories/Day

	DAY 1	2	3	4	5	6	7
WEEK ONE							
WEEK TWO							
WEEK THREE							

Record your weight *each day*

In the weeks that follow, you'll gradually increase your daily caloric intake; first to 1000, then to 1200 and then to 1800. After that you should stick to your proper maintenance level.

Obviously, in week four, you are simply adding 300 calories to the menu plan you followed during the first three weeks. The best way to do this is by adding single dishes to the lunch and dinner menus. Consult the Additional Recipes. Calories per serving are listed for each dish.

1000 Calories/Day

	DAY 1	2	3	4	5	6	7
WEEK FOUR							

1200 Calories/Day

	DAY 1	2	3	4	5	6	7
WEEK FIVE							

1800 Calories/Day

	DAY 1	2	3	4	5	6	7
WEEK SIX							

Finally, we've spoken about desired weight, and here is a table that will help you decide where you ought to be given your height and age:

Age

Height	TWENTIES	THIRTIES	FORTIES	FIFTIES	SIXTIES
Women 4'10"	97	102	106	109	111
5'1"	106	109	114	118	120
5'4"	114	118	122	127	129
5'7"	123	127	132	137	140
5'10"	134	138	142	146	147
Men 5'3"	125	129	130	131	130
5'6"	135	140	142	143	142
5'9"	149	153	155	156	155
6'0"	161	166	167	168	167
6'3"	176	181	183	184	180

Actual best weights will range widely depending upon the size of your frame. (From, for instance, 108 pounds for a small-framed woman to 138 for a large-framed woman, both of whom are 5'4" tall!)

Incidentally, recently I had an intense craving for something sweet. I had some frozen strawberries on hand, about a half cup. I thawed just enough so they'd still be firm. Then I put them in the blender, added ¼ cup of skim milk, a teaspoon of plain yogurt, a drop of vanilla extract, a packet of sugar substitute, and I pushed the button on the blender. Result? A fabulous strawberry shake. So for about 55 calories my craving for something sweet was satisfied. In the old days, I would have gone right to some junk food that has no nutritional benefit and is loaded with calories. Instead, I had protein, carbohydrate, fat, and fiber, and a minimal amount of calories. So start making up your own recipes and keep a file. You might want to write a book someday.

Freezer Tips

I use fresh vegetables and fruit in season whenever possible. I do, of course, use commercially frozen foods, but I try to do my own freezing as much as I can. If a particular fruit, such as figs (in season a short time), seems of really good quality, I wrap each piece individually in foil and label it with freezer tape—then into the freezer it goes. Figs do not have to be blanched before freezing. But remember, they are high in calories, so go easy.

Most fresh vegetables and fruits must be blanched before freezing. When I blanch them, I use a large spaghetti pot (a holdover from the old days), which has its own colander inside the pot. I fill the pot with about a gallon of water, adding a quarter of a cup of lemon juice. This helps to retain the color of whatever you are about to freeze. The blanching process begins when the water comes to a boil. Wash and trim vegetables, cutting off the hard stems of broccoli, for instance, using both the flowerets and stems. Boil three to four minutes. Drain. If you don't have a built-in colander, use a regular one. After draining, quickly dip the food into ice water. Transfer the food to freezer containers or freezer plastic bags, making sure they are airtight. Label, date, and freeze.

There are many fine books on freezing—for example, *Putting Food By* by Hertzberg, Vaughan, and Greene. A revised and enlarged paperback edition is published by Bantam Books. If you plan to do much freezing, I would advise you to read it.

Using commercially frozen foods is fine but read the ingredients on the package to make sure the vegetables and fruits are not packed in butter, sauces, or sugar-laden syrups.

I have also found that cooking frozen vegetables without adding water enhances the flavor and the vegetables turn out crispier. Enough water will come from the freezing process. The only advantage to adding water is to speed up the cooking process. Although it does take a little longer without the added water (about 20 minutes) it is worth it.

Do not thaw vegetables before cooking. They will come out mushy and tasteless.

- Juicy tomatoes bought in season can be washed, dried, and placed in plastic bags (uncooked) and frozen. This gives you fresh tasting tomatoes whenever you want them. The tomato skin peels off easily under cold water. Thaw, cook, and use for soups, stews, and so on.
- Fresh basil is available all year long. Simply cut the basil leaves off the stems, and line the leaves up on wax paper. Fold the paper, tape, and put into freezer. By

doing this you can use as much fresh basil as you want, without having to refreeze. The leaves peel easily off the wax paper as needed.

- Freeze egg yolks when making your egg white omelets, and give the yolks to a friend who bakes.
- The Lo-Cal dressing can be made in quantity and kept in the refrigerator for using. Just remember to stir ingredients before using.
- When the daily menu calls for half an apple, core and dice the other half, blanch, and store in freezer for recipes like Chicken with Raisins and Apples.
- When half a banana is called for, peel and wrap the other half in foil and freeze. This makes a delicious and refreshing taste treat.
- When one-half orange is called for, peel the other half and slice and freeze. Slightly thawed, this is wonderful with yogurt.
- When preparing something like Oven-Fried Chicken, where half a breast is one serving (because of breading ingredients and so on), remove the other ½ breast from oven in half the cooking time. Cool and wrap and freeze. On a day when you structure that recipe again, when reheating (after defrosting) the chicken will not be overcooked.
- Cool food quickly before freezing by putting food in a container in a pot of ice water. Putting hot food in refrigerator to cool raises the temperature in the refrigerator.
- Line a baking dish with heavy-duty foil. Put mixture you want to freeze in it (like stews, and so on), cover tightly with moisture-vapor proof wrap. Freeze. When frozen solid, remove the sealed-in foil ingredients, reseal, and return to freezer. This leaves the baking dish free for other baking jobs.
- Do not put strawberries for freezing in one plastic bag. You would have to thaw the entire bag before you could pry them apart. Simply line up the strawberries on a cookie or baking sheet, and place in freezer. When the strawberries are frozen firmly, remove each strawberry and pack in freezer container and return to freezer. Now, you can remove as many berries as you want without struggling.

- I like to extract the juice of lemons and pour it in ice cube trays and freeze. When frozen, simply remove cubes and transfer to plastic bag and return to freezer. This is wonderful for fresh lemonade or recipes that call for lemon juice. When doing this, I save the lemon peels (cutting off as much of the bitter white part as possible), mince the rind, freeze in plastic bag, and save for recipes requiring minced lemon rind.
- When freezing hamburger or veal patties, simply place a piece of freezer paper between each patty, so you can remove one at a time.
- Be sure to label and date everything you freeze. On several occasions I have thawed what I thought was chicken only to discover filet of sole. Certainly no big tragedy, but when chicken is called for, chicken is what I want.
- I have found the freezer to be an invaluable help when dieting; it allows me to use fresh vegetables and fruit which are out of season. Certainly you can buy frozen vegetables and fruit in your market, but why do that constantly when you can have them in your own freezer? You know what's in it because you prepared it. No hidden calories or artificial preservatives in *your* frozen foods.
- When preparing a recipe that calls for rice, make more than is required and freeze the remainder of the rice. Quickly-made dishes like Shrimp with Wine and Lemon Rind require only 10 minutes of cooking. Rice requires three times the amount of time to cook. Therefore, freeze rice in ¼ cup or ½ cup containers, remove, and steam. Saves lots of time and is just as delicious.
- I buy lots of small freezer containers to store things like chopped apples, lemon rinds, rice, chopped parsley, and so on, and label. This saves room in your freezer. The same can be done with heavy-duty foil, but I find the containers more convenient.

Additional Recipes

Green and Red Chicken Casserole

INGREDIENTS

1 *whole chicken breast, skinned and boned*
1 *small red pepper, cored and sliced*
1 *small green pepper, cored and sliced*
1 *cup mushrooms, sliced*
½ *cup chopped onion*
½ *cup skim milk*
¼ *cup dry white wine*
1 *tablespoon vegetable oil*

PREPARATION

Preheat oven to 350°. Cut chicken into small pieces. Saute the chicken, red and green peppers, mushrooms, and onions in a Teflon skillet, with the oil. Saute for only a short time, stirring until everything looks half done. Add the wine and simmer for about five minutes. Heat the skim milk. Set aside. Transfer all the ingredients into a 1-quart oven-proof casserole dish. Add the heated skim milk and mix. Cover and bake 30 minutes. Serves 2. Approximate calories: 250 per serving.

Carrots in Wine

INGREDIENTS

2 *cups grated carrots*
2 *tablespoons of dry white wine*
1 *tablespoon of diet margarine*
1 *teaspoon of lemon juice*
1 *teaspoon dehydrated onion flakes*
1 *tablespoon chopped chives*

PREPARATION

Preheat oven to 350°. Melt margarine in a pan and add the wine, lemon juice, onion flakes, and a dash of pepper. Heat for a few minutes. Spread grated carrots in a small oven-proof casserole dish. Pour the heated ingredients over the carrots. Bake for 20 minutes. Serves 2. Approximate calories: 65 per serving.

Baked Stuffed Potato

INGREDIENTS

$\frac{1}{2}$ *baked potato, medium size*
$\frac{1}{4}$ *cup cottage cheese*
Chives
Paprika

PREPARATION

Bake potato until done (350° for 1 hour). Slice potato in half and scoop out inside of one half, being careful not to break the skin. Return potato shell to the oven and bake until the shell is crisp. Mash the potato that has been scooped out. Add any flavoring you like—onion powder, garlic powder, etc. Add cottage cheese and whip until fluffy. Pour mixture back into potato shell. Top with chives or paprika. Return to oven and bake until reheated. Serves 1. Approximate calories: 95 per serving.

Asparagus Mozzarella Melt

INGREDIENTS

1 slice thin bread
½ ounce mozzarella
2 asparagus spears
1 tomato slice
¼ cup alfalfa sprouts

PREPARATION

Place tomato, asparagus, and alfalfa sprouts on top of thin bread. Place cheese on top. Broil until cheese melts and serve. Approximate calories: 115.

Fruit Compote

INGREDIENTS

¼ cup chopped apple
¼ cup diced orange
1 slice chopped pineapple
2 tablespoons plain yogurt

PREPARATION

Mix all ingredients. Serves 1. Approximate calories: 80.

Fast Food Potato Tacos

INGREDIENTS

2 medium-size potatoes
½ pound of lean ground beef
¼ wedge of lettuce, shredded
½ tomato, cut in 4 small wedges
Dash of tabasco sauce
1 slice of Lite-Line diet cheese, cut in 4 pieces
1 teaspoon black pepper
1 teaspoon corn oil
Minced onion
Dash of red pepper

PREPARATION

Cut potatoes in half, lengthwise. Scoop out center with a
spoon, leaving a shell with a thin layer of potato. Bake
potato shell in 350° oven for about 45 minutes, or until
crispy brown. Saute beef in a skillet with oil, minced onion,
black pepper, and red pepper. In each potato shell, place a
layer of beef, a generous amount of shredded lettuce, tabasco sauce, tomato wedges, and top with the diet cheese.
It's crunchy and delicious and satisfies that fast-food craving.
Calories per taco: 75

Basic Tomato Sauce

INGREDIENTS

2 pounds of tomatoes (about 5 cups)
1 tablespoon of vegetable oil
½ cup onion, chopped very fine
1 teaspoon minced garlic (optional)
½ teaspoon crushed red pepper
1 teaspoon chopped basil

PREPARATION

Wash and core tomatoes and cut in quarters. Heat oil in saucepan and, when hot, add onion and garlic, stirring until wilted. Add tomatoes and basil. Cover and let cook for 15 minutes. Remove from heat and let stand uncovered for 5 minutes, stirring the ingredients several times. Add crushed red pepper. Pour into the container of a food processor. This can also be done with an electric blender. Blend well. Return ingredients to saucepan and bring to a boil, stirring several times. And that's it.

This can be refrigerated or frozen in small freezer containers. I use this for just about anything that calls for tomato sauce, including cocktail sauce (adding a dash of horseradish), meat loaf, fish creole, and certainly over that occasional pasta dish.

Tuna Florentine

INGREDIENTS

8 ounces raw spinach (1 10-ounce frozen package)
1 ounce tuna
½ ounce cheddar cheese
2 tablespoons cream sauce

INGREDIENTS FOR CREAM SAUCE

6 ounces skim milk
1 tablespoon flour
1 teaspoon margarine

PREPARATION

Cook spinach. While spinach is cooking, begin to prepare cream sauce. Melt margarine, add flour, but do not brown. Mix well. Add a little cold milk. Mix. Heat mixture and slowly add cold milk. Stir and simmer until all of milk is added. If lumpy, put into blender. Drain spinach well. Place in casserole dish. Pour on 2 tablespoons of cream sauce. Sprinkle on tuna. Sprinkle on cheese. Bake at 350° for 30 minutes. Serve hot. Approximate calories: 125. To serve as an evening meal and increase the caloric amount, add 1 ounce tuna (30) and ½ ounce cheese (50). This increases the caloric amount to 205 calories.

Dilled Potatoes

INGREDIENTS

  2 peeled potatoes
  1 pat margarine
  1 teaspoon dill weed

PREPARATION

Cut peeled potatoes into 8 equal pieces. Put potatoes in pot, cover with water and boil until almost tender (15–20 mins.). Drain potatoes. Toss with margarine. Sprinkle dill weed on potatoes while tossing to coat evenly. Serve 4 pieces of potato. Approximate calories: 55 per serving.

Baked Mashed Potatoes

INGREDIENTS

  1 7-ounce potato (skinned)
  1 teaspoon margarine
  1 ounce skim milk

PREPARATION

Skin, slice, and boil potato for 10–15 minutes. After boiling, mash potato, add margarine and skim milk. Place mixture in small baking dish at 350° for 20 minutes. Serves 2. Approximate calories: 70 per serving.

Artichoke-Fruit Salad

INGREDIENTS

4 *drained artichoke hearts*
1/8 *cup low-calorie dressing*
1 *tablespoon red wine vinegar*
1/2 *teaspoon Worcestershire sauce*
1 1/2 *teaspoons dried parsley flakes*
1 1/2 *cups chopped iceberg lettuce*
1/2 *cups chopped curly endive*
1 *pink grapefruit, peeled and sectioned*

PREPARATION

Halve artichoke hearts. Combine the dressing, vinegar, Worcestershire sauce, and parsley flakes. Pour mixture over artichoke hearts, cover and chill 3–4 hours. In bowl, combine 3 types of lettuce. Pour liquid from artichoke hearts over lettuce, toss together. Serve: 3/4 cup mixed lettuce with dressing, 2 half-artichoke hearts, 4 grapefruit sections (sections from 1/4 grapefruit). Approximate calories: 50 per serving.

Tangy Chicken

INGREDIENTS

1 1/2 *pounds raw chicken breast*
12 *ounces tomato juice, salt-free*
1/4 *cup chopped celery*
1/2 *medium green pepper, chopped*
2 *tablespoons dehydrated onion flakes*
1 *teaspoon garlic powder*
1 *tablespoon Worcestershire Sauce*
3 *tablespoons red wine vinegar*
1/2 *lemon, cut into 1/4-inch rings*

PREPARATION

Combine in saucepan all ingredients except chicken. Simmer uncovered until reduced and slightly thickened. Place chicken in a shallow baking dish and cover with sauce, arranging lemon slices on top of chicken. Bake covered at 350° for 1 hour. (Bake uncovered for the last 15 minutes if you like it browned too.) Makes 2 6-ounce servings. Approximate calories: 315 per serving.

Beef Burgundy Rolls

INGREDIENTS

12 2-ounce slices raw roast beef

FOR STUFFING

2 slices thin bread, cubed
¼ cup diced mushrooms
⅛ cup minced onion
1 tablespoon red wine
1 tablespoon water
⅛ teaspoon sage
dash black pepper

GRAVY

1½ pats margarine
1½ tablespoons flour
¾ cup sliced mushrooms
¾ cup defatted beef broth
⅜ cup red wine
⅜ teaspoon garlic powder

PREPARATION (BEEF ROLLS)

Slice roast beef. Mix all stuffing ingredients in bowl. Put 1 tablespoon stuffing on each slice of beef, roll, put in baking pan sprayed with Pam. Put rolls in oven, bake 15 minutes at 350°. Pour half of mushroom gravy over beef rolls, bake for 30 minutes at 350° or until meat is done and stuffing is 140°. Serve 2 beef rolls with 1 ounce mushroom gravy on the side.

PREPARATION (GRAVY)

Toast flour lightly, mix with melted margarine to make roux. Add beef broth, stir until smooth and fairly thick. Stir in red wine, mushrooms, and garlic powder, and heat through.

Serves 6 (2 rolls per serving, with 2 ounces gravy). Approximate calories: 290 per serving.

Eggplant Special

INGREDIENTS

1 cup eggplant, sliced (⅛ inch)
½ cup cottage cheese
1 ounce part skim Mozzarella cheese
6 ounces tomato sauce
2 tablespoons chopped onion
1 teaspoon olive oil
oregano, garlic, marjoram

PREPARATION

Fry spices, onion, and olive oil in Teflon pan. Add tomato sauce and simmer. Slice eggplant into about 8 slices (⅛ inch thick). Place 4 slices in bottom of baking dish. Spread over cottage cheese and a little bit of the tomato sauce. Put on another 4 slices of eggplant. Pour over the rest of the tomato sauce. Sprinkle on top the Mozzarella cheese. Bake for ½ hour at 350°. Approximate calories: 330.

Chicken and Rice

INGREDIENTS

1½ pounds chicken legs
⅓ cup raw rice, 1 cup water
¼ cup celery, chopped
½ cup tomatoes, chopped
¼ cup green pepper, chopped
Spices: sage, paprika, marjoram, thyme, sweet basil

PREPARATION

Remove skin of chicken. Place chicken in casserole dish, on range burner. Add ¼ cup water, brown chicken on both sides for 5 minutes at low heat. Add rice, water, celery, tomatoes, green pepper, and spices. Bring heat to high and boil for 5–10 minutes. Add spices to taste. Lower heat to simmer for 45 minutes. Serves 2. Serving size (for 1): 6 ounces cooked meat, ½ cup cooked rice and vegetables. Approximate calories: 370 per serving.

Beef-Rice Casserole

INGREDIENTS

½ cup cooked rice
2½ ounces cooked beef
4½ tablespoons tomato sauce (see basic recipe)

PREPARATION

Prepare cooked rice (boil 20–25 minutes). Crumble and brown ground beef for 2–3 minutes. Place mixture in baking dish. Bake at 350° for 15–20 minutes. Serve with Basic Tomato Sauce (25 calories). Serves 1. Approximate calories: 275 per serving.

Easy Vegetable Soup

INGREDIENTS

1 quart water
1 cup diced celery
1 cup diced onion
1 cup diced tomatoes
3-ounce can tomato paste
1 cup carrots

PREPARATION

Add ingredients to water. Boil for ½ hour. Simmer for ½ hour. While cooking, add spices: garlic powder, bay leaf, thyme, oregano, and basil. The stock recipe may be used to enhance the flavor instead of water. Bits of chicken, beef, or turkey may also be used. If you wish, add 1 ounce of cooked lean meat to every quart of stock. Remember, the longer you boil the soup, the thicker the mixture, and the more calories per serving. Makes 4 to 5 6-ounce servings. Approximate calories: 50 per serving.

Baked Chicken with Mushrooms and Onions

INGREDIENTS

1½ pounds raw chicken breast (with bone)
½ teaspoon celery seed
½ teaspoon marjoram
½ cup chicken broth, defatted
1 cup fresh mushrooms
¼ cup onions, chopped

PREPARATION

Place chicken in a baking dish and sprinkle with celery seed and marjoram. Add the defatted chicken broth and bake, covered, in a 350° oven for 30 minutes. Baste occasionally. Then add the mushrooms and onions and continue baking for 20–30 minutes longer.

Stock Recipe

INGREDIENTS

4 ounces chicken, turkey, or small cubes of beef
½ onion
½ carrot
1 bay leaf
¼ teaspoon basil
⅛ teaspoon marjoram
4 whole peppercorns

PREPARATION

Take chopped chicken, turkey, or beef and put in pot of water (2 quarts). Chop onion and carrot fine. Add with spices to the meat and water. Cover. Simmer 4 hours. Cool to room temperature. Place stock in refrigerator and chill overnight. After discarding the fat that has hardened on top, warm stock until liquefied. Strain liquid. Remove any bones or pieces of meat. Sample the stock for flavor. If it is too weak it can be boiled longer to evaporate more liquid and concentrate the flavor. Makes 1 quart.

To Freeze: Pour ½ cup or 1 cup portions into covered containers. Freeze. Portion sizes depend on your uses and the number of people for whom you prepare meals. For individual servings, pour some stock into a refrigerator tray and freeze individual cubes. These cubes can be dropped into a plastic bag and removed when needed. Cubes can be added with water to vegetables for flavoring. A cup of stock can be defrosted and used to cook rice. A bit of stock can reheat leftover meats. And, of course, the stock is the base for making your vegetable soup.

Low-Calorie Salad Dressing

This dressing has negligible calories and can be used on salad or as a marinade.

INGREDIENTS

¼ cup unsweetened lemon juice
¼ cup red wine vinegar
1 teaspoon garlic
1 teaspoon vegetable oil
1 tablespoon chives
¼ tablespoon dill weed
½ tablespoon dry mustard
½ teaspoon black pepper

PREPARATION

Combine all ingredients. Refrigerate. Use 2 tablespoons of low-calorie salad dressing.

Chili Fried Chicken

INGREDIENTS

12 ounces chicken (1 breast split and skinned with bone)
1 tablespoon diet margarine
1 medium onion, peeled and minced
1 clove garlic, peeled and minced
1 fresh red chili, cut into strips
pepper to taste

PREPARATION

Heat diet margarine in Teflon frying pan. Saute the onion, garlic, and chili for 10 minutes. Put aside. Sprinkle the chicken with pepper and brown in skillet. Cover and cook over medium heat. After 20 minutes, uncover and scoop pepper, onions, and garlic mix (which should be dark brown) and place over chicken breast. Re-cover and cook for another 15 minutes, or until done. Serves 1. Approximate calories: 365.

Skillet Browned Potatoes

INGREDIENTS

> 4 medium potatoes, peeled
> 1 tablespoon safflower oil
> 1 tablespoon garlic powder
> Dash cayenne pepper
> ½ teaspoon curry powder
> ¼ teaspoon marjoram
> ¼ teaspoon thyme
> 1 tablespoon parsley flakes

PREPARATION

Cut each peeled potato in 6 equal pieces. Heat water, add potatoes, cover, and simmer about 10 minutes. Potatoes should be slightly undercooked. Drain potatoes and set aside. Heat oil in frying pan, add potatoes, and turn to coat with oil. Sprinkle spices evenly over potatoes. Cook potatoes until browned and tender. Serve 3 pieces of potato. Serves 6. Approximate calories: 75 per serving.

Potato Salad

INGREDIENTS

> 2 medium potatoes
> ¼ cup onion, chopped fine
> 2 tablespoons diet mayonnaise

PREPARATION

Scrub potatoes and peel. Boil 20 to 45 minutes, or until done. Dice potatoes. Mix potatoes with other ingredients. Chill 2 to 3 hours before serving. May garnish with paprika or parsley flakes. Serving size: ⅓ cup. Serves 4. Approximate calories: 70 per serving.

Basil Carrots

INGREDIENTS

    2 cups sliced carrots
    1 tablespoon melted diet margarine
    ¼ teaspoon basil

PREPARATION

Simmer carrots in water until tender and hot, and drain. Combine margarine and basil. Toss with carrots. Serve 1 cup. Serves 2. Approximate calories: 45 per serving.

Coleslaw

INGREDIENTS

    1½ cups white cabbage, chopped
    1½ cups red cabbage, chopped
    ½ cup carrots, sliced fine
    ⅛ teaspoon black pepper
    2 tablespoons diet mayonnaise

PREPARATION

Mix all ingredients together. Chill 2 to 3 hours before serving. Serving size: ½ cup. Serves 4. Approximate calories: 40 per serving.

Herb Baked Tomato

INGREDIENTS

½ cup bread crumbs (1 slice thin bread)
1½ tablespoons diet margarine
1¼ teaspoons garlic powder
1½ teaspoons ground coriander
1½ teaspoons ground cumin
4 tomatoes, 8 ounces each, halved

PREPARATION

Combine bread crumbs, margarine, and spices in small bowl, mixing well. Place tomatoes, cut side up, in baking dish. Top with bread crumb mixture. Bake at 150° for 35 to 45 minutes (or until tomatoes are soft and bread crumbs are lightly browned). Serve 1 tomato, 2 halves. Serves 4. Approximate calories: 55 per serving.

A Final Word on Exercise

Just the word exercise was enough to turn me into a defensive raging bull. "I hate exercise," I would say. It is just plain hype! Have you ever seen what those sneakers and matching outfits cost? Not to mention barbells and all that body pumping stuff.

I can still hear Gerry Musante giving me all kinds of information pertaining to the virtues of (here comes that word again) EXERCISE. I simply had a closed mind on the subject. Italians can be very, very stubborn.

I never felt exercise had anything to do with losing weight. After all, hadn't I lost pounds and pounds without ever doing a single pushup? Maybe I did gain it back, but that was due to gluttony, not because I hadn't run a marathon race that week.

As my knowledge about proper eating increased, so did the knowledge that being very, very stubborn can also be very, very dumb. I learned on a low calorie diet exercise could and did help me lose weight faster. Among other things I discovered that brisk walking decreased my appetite. Originally I tried the walking because I had hit a plateau and couldn't lose the weight as fast I wanted. Desperate to try anything, I decided to give exercise a shot.

After about a week of brisk walking (25 minutes after breakfast—the same after dinner) I felt calmer, more tranquil. I felt better and looked better, and, better still, I broke the plateau. So there had to be something in it after all. I started to do a little research and learned if one's metabolism is on the sluggish side, exercise could give it a permanent boost by 30 percent. Even the day after a binge exercise produced extra body heat and helped to burn off fat. It raises the metabolic rate and, of course, shows up on the scale.

I think the thing about exercise that always made me uncomfortable was thinking I had to do 100 pushups a day or some other *extreme* physical activity I simply couldn't handle or feel capable of.

I had spent my childhood shamefaced, unable to keep up with the class. There is nothing worse than a reformed uninformed. So take a walk . . . a brisk one . . . it's healthy, terrific for meeting new people, and you will love it.

Index

Index to Recipes

How's Your Health?

Bantam publishes a line of informative books, written by top experts to help you toward a healthier and happier life.

NEED MORE INFORMATION ON YOUR HEALTH AND NUTRITION?

Read the books that will lead you to
a happier and healthier life.

☐	23148	GETTING WELL AGAIN Simonton & Creighton	**$3.95**
☐	24246	DIET AND CANCER Kristin White	**$3.50**
☐	24775	UNDER THE INFLUENCE Milam & Ketcham	**$3.95**
☐	05024	THE JAMES COCO DIET James Coco & Marion Paone (A Hardcover Book)	**$13.95**
☐	23888	ARTHRITIC'S COOKBOOK Dong & Bank	**$3.50**
☐	20925	WHAT'S IN WHAT YOU EAT Will Eisner	**$3.95**
☐	34106	MY BODY, MY HEALTH Stewart & Hatcher (A Large Format Book)	**$11.95**
☐	24090	WOMEN AND THE CRISES IN SEX HORMONES G. Seamans	**$4.95**
☐	23335	GH-3-WILL IT KEEP YOU YOUNG LONGER H. Bailey	**$3.95**
☐	23827	THE HERB BOOK J. Lust	**$4.95**
☐	23767	HOPE AND HELP FOR YOUR NERVES C. Weekes	**$3.95**
☐	23818	PEACE FROM NERVOUS SUFFERING C. Weekes	**$3.95**
☐	24279	SIMPLE, EFFECTIVE TREATMENT OF AGORAPHOBIA C. Weekes	**$3.95**

Prices and availability subject to change without notice.